M000195871

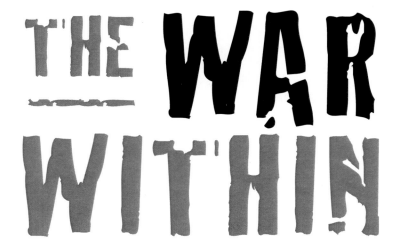

PREVENTING SUICIDE IN THE U.S. MILITARY

RAJEEV RAMCHAND | JOIE ACOSTA | RACHEL M. BURNS
LISA H. JAYCOX | CHRISTOPHER G. PERNIN

Prepared for the Office of the Secretary of Defense

Approved for public release; distribution unlimited

Center for Military Health Policy Research

A JOINT ENDEAVOR OF RAND HEALTH AND THE
RAND NATIONAL DEFENSE RESEARCH INSTITUTE

The research reported here was sponsored by the Office of the Secretary of Defense (OSD). The research was conducted jointly by the Center for Military Health Policy Research, a RAND Health program, and the Forces and Resources Policy Center, a RAND National Defense Research Institute (NDRI) program. NDRI is a federally funded research and development center sponsored by the OSD, the Joint Staff, the Unified Combatant Commands, the Navy, the Marine Corps, the defense agencies, and the defense Intelligence Community under Contract W74V8H-06-C-0002.

Library of Congress Control Number: 2011923237

ISBN: 978-0-8330-4971-1

Published 2011 by the RAND Corporation
1776 Main Street, P.O. Box 2138, Santa Monica, CA 90407-2138
1200 South Hayes Street, Arlington, VA 22202-5050
4570 Fifth Avenue, Suite 600, Pittsburgh, PA 15213-2665
RAND URL: http://www.rand.org/
To order RAND documents or to obtain additional information, contact
Distribution Services: Telephone: (310) 451-7002;
Fax: (310) 451-6915; Email: order@rand.org

Preface

Since late 2001, U.S. military forces have been engaged in conflicts around the globe, most notably in Iraq and Afghanistan. These conflicts have exacted a substantial toll on soldiers, marines, sailors, and airmen, and this toll goes beyond the well-publicized casualty figures. It extends to the stress that repetitive deployments can have on the individual servicemember and his or her family. This stress can manifest itself in different ways—increased divorce rates, spouse and child abuse, mental distress, substance abuse—but one of the most troubling manifestations is suicide, which is increasing across the U.S. Department of Defense (DoD). The increase in suicides among members of the military has raised concern among policymakers, military leaders, and the population at large. While DoD and the military services have had a number of efforts under way to deal with the increase in suicides among their members, the Assistant Secretary of Defense for Health Affairs asked the RAND National Defense Research Institute (NDRI) to do the following:

- Review the current evidence detailing suicide epidemiology in the military.
- Identify "best-practice" suicide-prevention programs.
- Describe and catalog suicide-prevention activities in DoD and across each service.
- Recommend ways to ensure that the activities in DoD and across each service reflect best practices.

This monograph, *The War Within: Preventing Suicide in the U.S. Military*, presents the results of that effort. The title reflects both the current struggle that DoD faces to confront an increasing number of suicides among military personnel and the internal, mental struggles that are so common among those who have died by or are contemplating suicide. This monograph was prepared specifically for health policy officials and suicide-prevention program managers (SPPMs) within DoD; however, the results should also be of interest to health policy officials within the U.S. Department of Veterans Affairs (VA), the U.S. Department of Health and Human Services, and the U.S. Congress.

This research was sponsored by the Assistant Secretary of Defense for Health Affairs and the Defense Centers of Excellence for Psychological Health and Traumatic

Brain Injury (DCoE). The research was conducted jointly by the RAND Center for Military Health Policy Research and the Forces and Resources Policy Center of the RAND National Defense Research Institute, a federally funded research and development center sponsored by the Office of the Secretary of Defense, the Joint Staff, the Unified Combatant Commands, the Navy, the Marine Corps, the defense agencies, and the defense Intelligence Community.

For more information on the Center for Military Health Policy Research, see http://www.rand.org/multi/military/ or contact the co-directors (contact information is provided on the web page). For more information on the Forces and Resources Policy Center, see http://www.rand.org/nsrd/about/frp.html or contact the director (contact information is provided on the web page).

Contents

Figures

Tables

Summary

Since late 2001, U.S. military forces have been engaged in conflicts around the globe, most notably in Iraq and Afghanistan. These conflicts have exacted a substantial toll on soldiers, marines, sailors, and airmen, and this toll goes beyond the well-publicized casualty figures. It extends to the stress that repetitive deployments can have on the individual servicemember and his or her family. This stress can manifest itself in different ways—increased divorce rates, spouse and child abuse, mental distress, substance abuse—but one of the most troubling manifestations is suicides, which are increasing across the U.S. Department of Defense (DoD). The increase in suicides among members of the military has raised concern among policymakers, military leaders, and the population at large. While DoD and the military services have had a number of efforts under way to deal with the increase in suicides among their members, they have also asked what more might be done and posed this question to the RAND National Defense Research Institute (NDRI). DoD asked NDRI to do the following:

- Review the current evidence detailing suicide epidemiology in the military.
- Identify "best-practice" suicide-prevention programs.
- Describe and catalog suicide-prevention activities in DoD and across each service.
- Recommend ways to ensure that the activities in DoD and across each service reflect best practices.

The RAND research team approached this task by reviewing all relevant policy and materials, as well as through key informant interviews with persons knowledgeable about suicide-prevention activities within DoD and with experts in the field of suicidology.

The Epidemiology of Suicide in the Military

The RAND research team took an epidemiological approach to answering questions of keen interest to DoD policymakers.

What Is the Suicide Rate in Military Services?

Suicide rates are typically reported in number of cases per 100,000 people. Figure S.1 shows the suicide rate among active-duty personnel for each military service and for DoD overall and reflects the published rate among active-duty military through 2008. It shows that, in 2008, the U.S. Marine Corps (USMC) and the U.S. Army have the highest rates (19.5 and 18.5, respectively), and the Air Force and the Navy have the lowest rates (12.1 and 11.6, respectively).

The figure also indicates that the suicide rate across DoD has been climbing, rising from 10.3 in 2001 to 15.8 in 2008, which represents about a 50-percent increase. The increase in the DoD suicide rate is largely attributable to a doubling of the rate in the Army. There is evidence that the suicide rate in DoD in calendar year (CY) 2007 was higher than those in CYs 2001 and 2002. There is also evidence that the rate in CY 2008 was higher than the annual rate between CYs 2001 and 2005 and higher than the average rate for CYs 2001 through 2008. Across services, there are significant differences in only the Army's suicide rate over time. Specifically, the Army suicide rates for CYs 2006 and 2007 were higher than in 2001 and 2004, and the rate in CY 2008 was higher than in it was between CY 2001 and CY 2005 and higher than the average rate for CYs 2001 through 2008.

Figure S.1
U.S. Department of Defense and Service Suicide Rates, 2001–2008

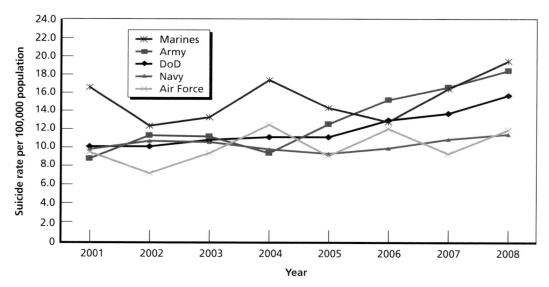

SOURCE: Mortality Surveillance Division, Armed Forces Medical Examiner.
RAND *MG953-S.1*

How Does the Military Suicide Rate Compare with That of the U.S. Population?

An important question is how the rate in the military compares with that of the general population. The estimated annual suicide rate in the general population for 2001–2006 hovers at around 10 per 100,000 (CDC, 2010), notably lower than that in DoD. But these populations are not necessarily comparable, because the military and the national population differ so much in terms of age, sex, and racial makeup and, in part, because the procedures for reporting suicide data also vary, both between states and regions and between the nation and DoD. To derive a comparable population, RAND researchers calculated an adjusted suicide rate for a synthetic national population having the same demographic profile as DoD personnel and as each service. Figure S.2 shows the results of comparing DoD with the comparable segment of the U.S. population for the years 2001–2006.[1] These results show that the suicide rate in the synthetic civilian population is both fairly constant and substantially higher than that in DoD. Of concern, however, is that the gap between DoD and the general population is closing. The most-pronounced increases in the DoD suicide rate occurred in 2007 and 2008, so, assuming that the national rate remains relatively stable in these years, the gap between the rate in DoD and the general population may be even narrower.

Figure S.2
Suicides in Adjusted U.S. Population and the U.S. Department of Defense

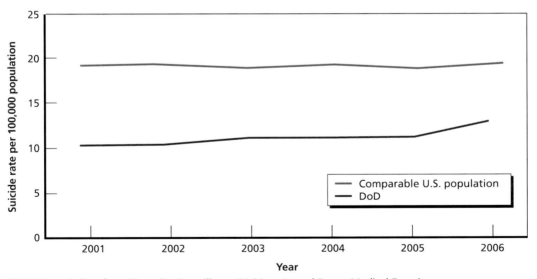

SOURCE: DoD data from Mortality Surveillance Division, Armed Forces Medical Examiner.
Comparable U.S. population data based on our estimates from CDC (2010).
RAND MG953-S.2

---

[1]   The most recent year for which data are available about suicides in the general U.S. population is 2006 (CDC, 2010).

Who Dies by Suicide in the Military?

One of the reasons that the synthetic population rates presented in Figure S.2 are higher than in the general population is because they represent the demographic profile of servicemembers in DoD, who are disproportionately male. In the United States, males are more likely to die by suicide than females—thus, the expected suicide rate based on this demographic characteristic alone is higher than for the country as a whole.

Who Is at Risk?

A review of the scientific literature revealed that those who are at a higher risk of dying by suicide fall into the following categories.

Prior Suicide Attempts. Although the majority of suicide deaths occur on individuals' first attempts and the majority of those who make a nonfatal suicide attempt do not go on to die by suicide, a prior suicide attempt is the strongest predictor of subsequent death by suicide (Isometsa and Lonnqvist, 1998, Harris and Barraclough, 1997).

Mental Disorders. Certain mental disorders that carry an increased risk of suicide, such as schizophrenia, are of minimal concern to the military because many learning, psychiatric, and behavioral disorders are cause for rejection at enlistment and during training. However, the continuing deployments of U.S. military personnel to Iraq and Afghanistan have highlighted the emergence of specific mental health concerns that are relevant to this population: depression and anxiety disorders (including posttraumatic stress disorder, or PTSD). The Institute of Medicine (IOM) estimates that approximately 4 percent of those with depression will die by suicide (Goldsmith et al., 2002), and, though the same figure is not yet known for those with PTSD, community-based surveys indicate that persons with PTSD are more likely than those without the disorder to report past suicide attempts and ideation (Kessler, Borges, and Walters, 1999; Sareen et al., 2005; Farberow, Kang, and Bullman, 1990).

Substance-Use Disorders. People with substance-use disorders and heavy users of alcohol and other drugs face an increased risk for suicide, depending on the presence of a disorder and the type of drug that they use. While drug use is not prevalent in the military largely due to routine screening, approximately 20 percent of servicemembers report heavy alcohol use (drinking five or more drinks per typical drinking occasion at least once per week) (Bray and Hourani, 2007).

Head Trauma/Traumatic Brain Injury (TBI). Evidence also indicates that persons with concussions, cranial fractures, or cerebral contusions or traumatic intracranial hemorrhages had higher rates of suicide mortality than the general population (Teasdale and Engberg, 2001; Simpson and Tate, 2002, 2005). TBI is of particular concern among deployed military personnel who may sustain blast or other concussive injuries as a result of an explosion or blast of an improvised explosive device (IED).

Those Suffering from Hopelessness, Aggression and Impulsivity, and Problem-Solving Deficits. Although mental and substance-use disorders are common among those who die by suicide, the majority of those with such disorders do not die this way (Harris and Barraclough, 1997; Wilcox, Conner, and Caine, 2004; Goldsmith et al., 2002). Researchers have conducted studies to see how persons with the same mental disorders differ with respect to a history of suicide attempts and death by suicide. Those with high levels of hopelessness are at increased risk, and there is some evidence that higher levels of aggression and impulsivity, as well as those with problem-solving deficits, are also at increased risk for suicide (McMillan et al., 2007; Mann et al., 1999; Rudd, Rajab, and Dahm, 1994).

Life Events, Precipitating Events, and Triggers. There is some concern about specific life events (e.g., death of family member, relationship problems) among servicemembers who die by suicide. While there is some evidence suggesting that particular life events differentially increase the risk of suicide (Luoma and Pearson, 2002), such studies have not been conducted among military personnel. Most of the scientific literature suggests that it is the interaction with underlying vulnerabilities, such as behavioral health problems, that influence a suicidal response to these relatively common events (Yen et al., 2005; Joiner and Rudd, 2000).

Firearm Access. Consistent evidence indicates that availability of firearms correlates positively with suicide (Matthew Miller, Lippmann, et al., 2007; Matthew Miller, Azrael, et al., 2006). Military personnel have access to firearms, particularly when deployed, and are more likely to own a personal gun than are members of the general population (Hepburn et al., 2007). Thus, military personnel who are considering suicide are more likely to have access to a firearm, one of the most lethal ways people can kill themselves.

Suicides of Others and Reporting of Suicides. For youth and young adults, there is evidence of contagion—that a suicide may lead to subsequent suicides (Insel and Gould, 2008). There is evidence of suicide clusters primarily among teens (Gould, 1990; Gould, Wallenstein, and Kleinman, 1990; Gould, Wallenstein, Kleinman, et al., 1990), though such clusters generally account for less than 5 percent of youth suicides (Insel and Gould, 2008). Media reporting of suicides, particularly coverage that lasts for a long time, is featured prominently, and is covered extensively in newspapers, is also associated with increases in suicide (Gould, 2001), though adhering to media guidelines on such reporting can mitigate any possible contagion (Pirkis et al., 2006).

Best Practices

RAND researchers reviewed a wide range of prevention programs, assessing them for their application to the military. These programs included universal programs that target entire populations and selected or indicated programs that focus on specific groups at high risk. They also considered self-care (i.e., maintaining one's personal health), making the environment safer, and *postvention*, which refers to the way an organization or media outlet treats a death by suicide. Taken together, these programs form a continuum of prevention activities ranging from programs delivered on a broad scale at a relatively small cost per person to treatment programs delivered to few at high expense.

The challenge in identifying best practices for suicide prevention is the lack of data on the effectiveness of programs. A best practice for suicide prevention would be one supported by empirical evidence showing that it causally reduced suicides. Currently, only a handful of programs would meet this definition. The bulk of the strong evidence about effectiveness concentrates at the selected prevention end of the spectrum, focusing on interventions or treatments for those who have displayed past suicidal behavior or those deemed to be at increased risk for suicide (see Chapter Three).

Universal programs with specific suicide-prevention activities generally fall into two categories: those that raise awareness and teach skills and those that provide screening and referral for mental health problems and suicidal behavior. Selected programs also fall into two categories: those that target groups at high risk by virtue of a known risk factor (e.g., mental illness) and those that work directly with suicide attempters who come to the attention of health providers because of their suicidal behavior. Environmental safety programs attempt to identify the means by which people kill themselves in a particular population and then to make these means less available. Examples of such initiatives include policies that restrict access to firearms to prevent self-inflicted gunshot wounds, use of blister packs (which require an individual to extract each pill from a sealed plastic pocket) for lethal medications to prevent intentional overdoses, bridge safeguards to prevent fatal falls, and constructing shower-curtain rods so as to prevent fatal hangings. Postvention efforts primarily have to do with establishing rules and responsibilities for community organizations following a suicide. Postvention also includes training the media on guidelines for proper reporting of suicides to reduce the possibility of imitative suicides. Such training includes not glorifying the death or describing the means by which suicide victims ended their lives.

Our assessment of these various programs indicates that promising practices exist, but much remains unknown about what constitutes a best practice. Our assessment of the literature and conversations with experts in the field indicate that a comprehensive suicide-prevention program should include the following six practices:

1. *Raise awareness and promote self-care.* One clear finding that emerges from the literature is that a focus on skill building may be important at all stages of prevention. Reducing known risk factors, such as substance abuse and mental health problems, is often included as one aspect of integrated approaches.

2. *Identify those at high risk.* Selected or indicated prevention is a fundamental component of a public health approach to disease prevention and is predicated on identifying those at higher risk. Thus, a comprehensive suicide-prevention program should have means by which this may occur, such as screening for

mental health problems, one of the strongest risk factors for suicide, in primary care or through the use of gatekeepers.

3. *Facilitate access to quality care.* Access to quality behavioral health care is an integral component of many suicide-prevention programs. Past research highlights that a number of barriers obstruct such access, including some barriers that are specific to the military. Although reducing barriers to mental health care has not been specifically correlated with reducing suicides except as part of broad, integrated programs, facilitating access to effective care will help ensure that those at increased risk will receive quality care and thus reduce suicides.

4. *Provide quality care.* The types of interventions with the strongest empirical support for effectively preventing suicide involve quality mental health treatment and specific interventions focused on suicidality. The need to ensure quality of behavioral health services is a critical and often overlooked component of suicide prevention.

5. *Restrict access to lethal means.* There is evidence that restricting access to lethal means is an effective way to prevent suicide. Universal means restriction might be difficult in the U.S. military, with weapons readily available to deployed soldiers. However, selected or indicated programs that limit gun availability to persons deemed to be at high risk of suicide should be considered.

6. *Respond appropriately.* Given evidence of possible imitative suicides, suicide-prevention programs must have in place a strategy for responding to a suicide. Such a strategy should focus on how details of the suicide are communicated in the media, as well as how the information is passed on to groups to which the deceased individual belonged (e.g., classmates, colleagues, military unit).

Suicide Prevention in the U.S. Department of Defense and Across the Services

Each of the services is engaged in a variety of suicide-prevention activities. For each service, we amassed information on the underlying philosophy (stated or not) behind that service's suicide-prevention program, and a description of programs and initiatives along with information about how each service supports suicide-prevention activities (i.e., official documentation bearing on suicide, organizations responsible for suicide prevention, how suicide-prevention programs and initiatives are funded).

Suicide Prevention in the U.S. Department of Defense

There are five cross-service suicide-prevention initiatives sponsored by DoD. First, the DoD Suicide Prevention and Risk Reduction Committee is a committee of key stakeholders, including each service's suicide-prevention program manager (SPPM), that meets monthly to provide input on policy, develop joint products, and share information. Second, in 2008, the Defense Centers of Excellence for Psychological Health and Traumatic Brain Injury (DCoE) began funding the Real Warriors Campaign, a public education initiative to address the stigma of seeking psychological care and treatment. Third, in 2009, DoD established a congressionally directed DoD Task Force on the Prevention of Suicide by Members of the Armed Forces, which is expected to release its findings in the summer or fall of 2010. Fourth, in 2008, all services began conducting surveillance on suicide events (suicides and attempts or ideation that results in hospitalization or evacuation) using the same surveillance tool: the Department of Defense Suicide Event Report (DoDSER). Finally, since 2002, DoD has sponsored an annual suicide-prevention conference; in 2009 and 2010, the conference was jointly sponsored by DoD and the U.S. Department of Veterans Affairs (VA).

Suicide Prevention in the Army

The Army's current approach to suicide prevention revolves around programs that encourage "soldiers to take care of soldiers" and those that offer a holistic approach to promote resiliency. This information is dispensed primarily through public awareness campaigns and training and education offered to both leaders and soldiers. The message is exemplified by the Army's Ask, Care, Escort (ACE) program that serves as the cornerstone of most current suicide-prevention efforts. Resiliency programs are offered to persons before deploying and upon returning from deployment. New approaches to facilitate access to care include public-awareness campaigns designed to eliminate stigma associated with seeking behavioral health-care treatment and locating behavioral health-care professionals in nontraditional settings, such as primary care and in theater.

In the past, the Deputy Chief of Staff for Army Personnel (G-1) provided the funding required for the Army Suicide Prevention Program (ASPP) to execute its suicide-prevention mission. However, since the establishment of the Suicide Prevention Task Force in March 2009 and the added emphasis placed on suicide prevention, there is a dedicated line of funding in the Army's fiscal year (FY) 2011 budget for suicide prevention and some elements that support it. Nonetheless, suicide-prevention activities are developed, managed, and run across multiple organizations within the Army, including the suicide-prevention program office within G-1 and the U.S. Army Center for Health Promotion and Preventive Medicine (CHPPM),[2] Deputy Chief of Staff for Army Operations (G-3), and from such senior leaders as the Vice Chief of Staff of the Army.

Suicide Prevention in the Navy

The Navy's approach to suicide prevention is guided by a model that sees stress on a continuum and in which suicide represents an extreme endpoint on the continuum.

---

[2]   CHPPM is in the process of changing to the U.S. Army Public Health Command (see APHC, 2010).

The model emphasizes early intervention to prevent and manage stress, particularly in the face of challenging life events (e.g., relationship or financial difficulties). This information is conveyed via media campaigns and educational programs and trainings, the cornerstone of which is Operational Stress Control. The Navy also places behavioral health-care providers in nontraditional settings, such as providing community-based outreach coordinators for reservists or placing psychologists on aircraft carriers.

The majority of suicide-prevention initiatives in the Navy are funded by the responsible agencies and organizations, though there will be some dedicated funding for suicide prevention in FY 2010. The Navy SPPM serves in this capacity on a part-time basis.

Suicide Prevention in the Air Force

The Air Force approach to preventing suicide is based on initiating cultural changes in attitudes and actions pertaining to suicide and implementing these changes through the highest-ranking Air Force officials. The program is comprised of 11 tenets outlined in an Air Force pamphlet (AFPAM 44-160). These tenets require training and education for all airmen, but also include policies and procedures for monitoring individuals for suicidal behavior following an investigative interview and, in these cases, protect the confidentiality of those receiving treatment from a psychotherapist. The Air Force program also established entities at the installation, major command (MAJCOM), and Air Force levels called the Integrated Delivery System (IDS), which is a conglomeration of Air Force organizations engaged in suicide prevention and related activities that organize and coordinate prevention programs and are guided by the Community Action Information Boards (CAIBs). Guidance to Air Force behavioral health-care providers on assessing and managing suicidal risk is provided through a published guide created by the Air Force and a one-time training that was offered in 2007 with an accompanying plan for sustainment via chain-teaching. There is published evidence to suggest that the implementation of the Air Force Suicide Prevention Program (AFSPP) was associated with a 33-percent risk reduction in suicide (Knox et al., 2003). It has been reviewed by the National Registry of Evidence-Based Programs and Practices, which found that research methods were strong enough to support these claims (SAMHSA, 2010).

Agencies and organizations are responsible for using internal funds to support their responsibilities outlined for that organization, though there is also a full-time Air Force SPPM and a dedicated stream of funding for suicide prevention.

Suicide Prevention in the Marine Corps

The Marine Corps approach to suicide prevention relies primarily on programs in which members of the USMC community are trained to identify and refer marines at risk for suicide to available resources (e.g., a commander, chaplain, mental health professional). The core of the Marine Corps approach occurs via education and training that all marines receive annually both during their required martial-arts training and from their local commands. Special training is offered to all new marines (officers and enlisted) and their drill instructors, front-line leaders (noncommissioned officers [NCOs] and lieutenants), and civilian employees who have regular direct contact with a large proportion of the force. Public-awareness messages disseminated via videos, posters, and brochures aim to reduce the stigma of getting help. Behavioral health providers and chaplains who serve marines were also offered a one-time voluntary training on assessing and managing suicidal risk. Finally, there is also a program to support marines before, after, and during deployment, and behavioral health professionals are embedded in infantry regiments to increase marines' access to behavioral health services.

Agencies and organizations are responsible for using internal funds to support the responsibilities outlined for that organization, though there is also a full-time Marine Corps SPPM and four full-time staff dedicated to suicide prevention at USMC Headquarters.

Conclusions

We assessed how each of the services was performing across the six domains of a comprehensive suicide-prevention program. Their performance is outlined in Table S.1.

Raise Awareness and Promote Self-Care

The services use media campaigns, training and educational courses, and messages from key personnel to raise awareness and promote self-care. Most of the messages conveyed focus on raising awareness, which has limited evidence of creating behavior change. Across services, there are fewer messages disseminated with respect to promoting self-care; those that do exist are generally geared toward deploying personnel or those returning from deployments. Few programs teach strategies to help servicemembers build skills that would help them care for themselves, including the ability to self-refer when needed.

Identify Those at High Risk

The Army, Navy, and Marine Corps generally rely on "gatekeepers" to identify people at increased risk for suicide and actively refer those in distress to follow-up care. There is insufficient evidence to date indicating that these training programs are effective at reducing suicides. An alternative strategy for identifying those at high risk of suicide is to monitor the aftermath of high-risk events. The Air Force does this by monitoring those under investigation, and the Army, Navy, and Air Force all have programs that attempt to monitor servicemembers after deployment to mitigate potentially negative consequences of deployment. The Army and Air Force also have programs that pro

Table S.1
Assessment of Suicide-Prevention Activities Across Services

Goal	Army	Navy	Air Force	Marines
Raise awareness and promote self-care	Primarily awareness campaigns, with fewer initiatives aimed at promoting self-care			
Identify those at risk	Expansive but rely mostly on gatekeepers	Mostly rely on gatekeepers	Investigation policy	Mostly rely on gatekeepers
Facilitate access to quality care	Stigma addressed primarily by locating behavioral health care in nontraditional settings			
	No policy to assuage privacy or professional concerns		Limited privilege	No policy
	No education about benefits of accessing behavioral health care			
Deliver quality care	Not considered in domain of suicide prevention		Past efforts exist with a sustainment plan	Past efforts exist, but not sustained
Restrict access to lethal means	No current policies exist		Limited guidance	No policy
Respond appropriately	Personnel/teams available, but limited guidance			

mote mental health screening in primary care. Only the Air Force and Marines have trained behavioral health-care professionals in suicide risk assessment and management, which some experts we interviewed considered to be a promising practice.

Programs aimed at identifying those at high risk should be based on research that discerns those at high risk; the Army is actively pursuing research that could provide information about Army-specific risk factors, and the Air Force has a consultation tool by which any Air Force commander can request an investigation to assess his or her unit's well-being.

Facilitate Access to Quality Care

Across the services, most of the initiatives in place to facilitate access to quality care fall under the domain of eliminating stigma: Initiatives that raise awareness about suicide and promote self-care can reduce stigma, as can locating behavioral health care in nontraditional settings, including in primary care and in theater. There are fewer initiatives focused on assuaging servicemembers' career and privacy concerns, and there are few initiatives under the purview of suicide prevention that seek to dispel myths about the ineffectiveness of behavioral health care, both of which are well-established barriers to such care among military personnel, though such information is conveyed in the Air Force's and Marine Corps' annual training. In addition, the recently launched Real Warriors campaign does begin to fill this gap.

Provide Quality Care to Those in Need

Providing quality care is a fundamental component of suicide prevention. It was beyond the scope of the current research project to evaluate the quality of care offered by behavioral health-care providers, though only the Air Force and Marine Corps made us aware of programs aimed at improving the skills of behavioral health-care providers with respect to assessing and managing suicidal patients. However, in both services, these programs were one-time offerings with no plan for additional training. But the Air Force teaches this material informally in its internship and residency programs, as well as by providing a manual, training videos, and assessment measures to each clinic.

Restrict Access to Lethal Means

Across the services, there are no known specific policies in place in which access to lethal means is restricted for the purposes of reducing suicides, either universally or for those at increased or imminent risk of suicide. The Air Force provides limited guidance to leaders on means restriction when managing personnel in severe distress.

Respond Appropriately to Suicides and Suicide Attempts

Each service has a team or personnel on whom leaders can call to assist them after a suicide specifically or traumatic event more generally. However, no policies or guidance provide details on what should be done if and when a unit experiences the loss of one of its own to suicide.

Recommendations

We make 14 recommendations pertinent to all services:

1. *Track suicides and suicide attempts systematically and consistently.* The recent initiatives to use the DoDSER and establish a common nomenclature across all services will help ensure that communication on suicide is consistent within DoD and foster information sharing between the services. However, this will also require that the services and each installation are using the same criteria for determining who requires a DoDSER.

2. *Evaluate existing programs and ensure that new programs contain an evaluation component when they are implemented.* Evaluation provides a basis for decision-making and helps ensure that resources are used effectively and to achieve anticipated outcomes. Current initiatives should be evaluated, and an evaluation plan should be a required component of any new initiative.

3. *Include training in skill building, particularly help-seeking behavior, in programs and initiatives that raise awareness and promote self-care.* Most universal prevention programs in the services focus on raising awareness about suicide, provide

resources to which a servicemember can turn when he or she (or someone he or she knows) is feeling suicidal, and may include messages about the importance of peer gatekeepers. There is no evidence to indicate that any of these strategies is effective on its own. A limitation of these kinds of programs is that they do not teach the skills that servicemembers may need to refer themselves to behavioral health professionals or chaplains.

4. *Define the scope of what is relevant to preventing suicide, and form partnerships with the agencies and organizations responsible for initiatives in other areas.* Behavioral health problems (e.g., mental disorders, harmful substance-using behaviors) are risk factors for suicide, and prevention efforts across all of these domains have the potential to affect suicides in DoD. Thus, it is important that suicide-prevention programs within each service create partnerships with the organizations responsible for these other areas to ensure consistent messaging, create jointly sponsored projects, and avoid duplication.

5. *Evaluate gatekeeper training.* The services rely heavily on gatekeeper training, a prevention technique for which there is no evidence of effectiveness (though for which there have been few evaluations). Gatekeeper training is intuitively appealing because it can reach a wide number of people, and the use of non-military gatekeepers might help reduce the stigma associated with recognizing and referring a peer in uniform. On the other hand, it may send the message that suicide is always another person's problem, and some individuals will not be good gatekeepers and should not be relied on to serve in this capacity. Servicemembers may also not intervene out of fear that their actions could jeopardize a fellow servicemember's military career. Evaluation of gatekeeper programs is needed to help clarify these issues.

6. *Develop prevention programs based on research and surveillance; selected and indicated programs should be based on clearly identified risk factors specific to military populations and to each service.* Most services produce reports that provide descriptive information about servicemembers who have killed themselves but cannot identify the factors that actually place individuals at risk of killing themselves, which would require a well-defined control group. Identifying risk factors is critical in the development of selected and indicated prevention programs, which are important components of a public health approach to suicide prevention.

7. *Ensure that continuity of services and care are maintained when servicemembers or their caregivers transition between installations in a process that respects servicemembers' privacy and autonomy.* Because military personnel transition frequently between installations and commands, as well as between active and reserve status, it is important that they know of the resources available at each new command. For those receiving formal behavioral health care or counseling from a chaplain, efforts should be made to help ensure that the servicemember

continues to receive the necessary care when he or she (or his or her caregiver) transfers. We recommend that patients themselves manage this process, with support from behavioral health-care providers and chaplains. For example, behavioral health-care providers and chaplains should provide clients moving to a new installation with the contact information for analogous resources at the new installation, encourage their clients to make appointments soon after arriving, and occasionally check in with them.

8. *Make servicemembers aware of the benefits of accessing behavioral health care and specific policies and repercussions for accessing such care, and conduct research to inform this communication.* Military personnel share a widespread belief that behavioral health care is ineffective and a concern that seeking behavioral health care could harm their career. There are no explicit policies with respect to repercussions across the services for accessing this care. Research is needed to discern the effect that seeking behavioral health care has on a servicemember's military career.

9. *Make servicemembers aware of the different types of behavioral health caregivers available to them, including information on caregivers' credentials, capabilities, and the confidentiality afforded by each.* The behavioral health-care workforce in the military is diverse and varies with respect to education, licensing, and certification or credentialing. Each service also relies heavily on chaplains who are embedded in military units and often serve as front-line responders for persons under psychological or emotional duress. Educating military personnel about the differences among referral specialists with respect to each professional's credentials and professional capabilities is important. Also, each provider is responsible for knowing what type of care he or she is capable of providing and to refer as appropriate. Confidentiality is noted to be a specific barrier to care among this population and is not uniform across providers: For example, chaplains offer total confidentiality, but command staff has access to information about servicemembers' access of professional mental health services (i.e., care offered in a clinical setting). Servicemembers should therefore also be made aware of the confidentiality afforded by different organizations and individuals.

10. *Improve coordination and communication between caregivers and service providers.* Those who offer behavioral health care should work as a team to ensure that the emotional well-being of those for whom they care is maintained. There were conflicting reports about the relationship between these professionals on military bases. For example, some interviewees reported open communication and collegiality between chaplains and behavioral health-care providers, while others reported a more acrimonious relationship. Improved communication and collaboration between professionals helps create a trustworthy hand-off to ensure that individuals do not fall through the cracks when going from one form of care to another.

11. *Assess whether there is an adequate supply of behavioral health-care professionals and chaplains available to servicemembers.* Effective suicide prevention in the military will rely on persons accessing quality behavioral health care and counseling. Messages promoting these resources assume a capacity of providers and chaplains who can deliver quality care to those who request it. There appears to be a need for research to address this concern: Chaplains, for example, reported that they thought they were understaffed, though they did not have empirical basis for this assumption. There is also a shortage of behavioral health-care providers in the United States generally, and DoD has faced challenges in recruiting and retaining adequately trained behavioral health-care providers.

12. *Mandate training on evidence-based or state-of-the-art practices for behavioral health generally and in suicide risk assessment specifically for chaplains, health-care providers, and behavioral health-care professionals.* Programs that promote behavioral health-care providers and chaplains often operate under the assumption that these individuals are sufficiently trained in assessing and managing suicidal patients. Unfortunately, this assumption may not be valid: Few providers are adequately trained in effective ways to assess risk and manage patients at varying levels of risk. Guides do exist that, while not evidence-based, offer helpful guidelines to providers. Both the Air Force and Marine Corps have independently conducted training, but these efforts were one-time occurrences with no future plans. There is also an implicit assumption that these professionals are trained to provide more general high-quality care and counseling. Unfortunately, research from the civilian sector indicates that the provision of quality care for behavioral health is not universal across mental health-care providers, and there is no reason to think that services in the military are any different. There is almost no evidence on the quality of counseling offered by chaplains. The quality of mental health care and counseling offered in DoD is unknown, and efforts to improve quality, such as training providers in evidence-based practice, are not integrated into the system of mental health care offered in DoD treatment facilities. Training all health-care providers on mental health awareness and quality behavioral health care is also an important component of provider training.

13. *Develop creative strategies to restrict access to lethal means among military servicemembers or those indicated to be at risk of harming themselves.* A comprehensive suicide-prevention strategy should have considered ways to restrict access to the means by which servicemembers could try to end their own lives. Due to the prevalence of firearms as a means by which military servicemembers die by suicide, initiatives to restrict access to firearms should be considered. Although restricting firearms among military personnel seems daunting or even impossible, there is some precedent for such policies in both the Veterans Health Administration (VHA) and DoD. In particular, selected or indicated

prevention strategies may include restricting access to firearms specifically among those identified to be at risk of harming themselves.

14. *Provide formal guidance to commanders about how to respond to suicides and suicide attempts.* Responding to a suicide appropriately not only can help acquaintances of the suicide victim grieve but also can prevent possible imitative suicides, as well as serve as a conduit to care for those at high risk. Across services, there is no direct policy regarding appropriate ways in which a leader should respond to a suicide within his or her unit. Fear of imitative suicides may also hinder many leaders from openly discussing suicides in their units. There also needs to be guidance for leaders to help care for and integrate servicemembers back into units who have made suicide attempts or expressed suicidal ideation, as there are anecdotal reports of servicemembers being ostracized or ridiculed after seeking behavioral health care or having been treated for suicidal behavior. Not only does this increase the risk of another suicide attempt, but it also creates a hostile and stigmatizing environment for others in the unit who may be under psychological or emotional duress.

Suicide is a tragic event, though the research suggests that it can be prevented. The recommendations represent the ways in which the best available evidence suggests that some of these untimely deaths could be avoided.

Acknowledgments

The authors would like to acknowledge several individuals who helped in preparing this manuscript. Within the Department of Defense, the study project monitors provided excellent guidance and support. Specifically, at the Defense Centers of Excellence for Psychological Health and Traumatic Brain Injury, CDR Janet Hawkins, and, at the Office of the Assistant Secretary of Defense for Health Affairs, COL Robert Ireland. Also at the Office of the Assistant Secretary of Defense for Health Affairs, Lucinda Frost was an extremely valuable resource. This research relied on key informant interviews, and we thank all of those who volunteered their time and expertise (those who agreed to have their names listed are presented in Tables 1.1 and 1.2 in Chapter One). In addition to our key informant interviews, all of those who participated in the DoD Suicide Prevention and Risk Reduction Committee during our study period were helpful, including Lt. Col. Mitchell Luchansky, Walter Morales, CAPT Joyce Lapa, Lynne Oetjen-Gerdes, Gregory Gahm, Janet Kemp, Mark Reger, LTC Mary Hull, and CDR Jerry O'Toole. Many individuals at RAND were instrumental in helping prepare this monograph, including Terri Tanielian, and Susan Hosek, Jerry Sollinger, Craig Martin, Kristin Lang, Laura Miller, Kevin Feeney, and Emily Bever. Finally, we acknowledge our reviewers: at RAND, Grant Marshall; at the National Institute of Mental Health, Jane Pearson; and at Yale University, Annette Beautrais.

Abbreviations

AAS	American Association of Suicidology
ACE	Ask, Care, Escort
ACT	Ask, Care, Treatment
AF/A1	Deputy Chief of Staff for Manpower and Personnel
AF/A3/5	Deputy Chief of Staff, Air, Space and Information Operations, Plans and Requirements
AF/A4/7	Air Force Deputy Chief of Staff for Logistics, Installations and Mission Support
AF/CC	Air Force Chief of Staff
AF/CCC	Air Force Command Chief Master Sergeant
AF/HC	Air Force Chaplain Corps
AFI	Air Force instruction
AF/JA	Air Force Judge Advocate
AFMS	Air Force Medical Service
AF/RE	Air Force Reserve
AF/SE	Air Force Safety
AF/SG	Air Force Surgeon General
AFPAM	Air Force pamphlet
AFSPP	Air Force Suicide Prevention Program
AGR	Active Guard and Reserve

AID LIFE	ask, intervene immediately, do not keep it a secret, locate help, inform the chain of command of the situation, find someone to stay with the person now, and expedite
AIDS	acquired immune deficiency syndrome
AIRS	Automated Inspection Reporting System
AKO	Army Knowledge Online
AMEDD	Army Medical Department
APS	Army Posture Statement
AR	Army regulation
ARNG	Army National Guard
ASAP	Army Substance Abuse Program
ASER	Army Suicide Event Report
ASIST	Applied Suicide Intervention Skills Training
ASPP	Army Suicide Prevention Program
ASPTF	Army Suicide Prevention Task Force
BUMED	Bureau of Medicine and Surgery
CACO	casualty assistance calls officer
CAIB	Community Action Information Board
CAMS	Collaborative Assessment and Management of Suicidality
CASE	Chronological Assessment of Suicide Events
CDC	Centers for Disease Control and Prevention
CHPC	Community Health Promotion Council
CHPPM	U.S. Army Center for Health Promotion and Preventive Medicine
CISD	Critical Incident Stress Debriefing
CO	commanding officer
CONUS	continental United States
COSC	Combat Operational Stress Control

CSC	combat stress control
CSCP	combat stress control prevention
CSCR	combat stress control restoration
CSF	Comprehensive Soldier Fitness
CT	cognitive therapy
CTS	called to serve
CY	calendar year
DA	Department of the Army
DAPE-HRI	Office of the Deputy Chief of Staff, G-1, Army Values
DBT	dialectical behavior therapy
DCoE	Defense Centers of Excellence for Psychological Health and Traumatic Brain Injury
DEERS	Defense Enrollment Eligibility Reporting System
DMDC	Defense Manpower Data Center
DoD	U.S. Department of Defense
DoDSER	Department of Defense Suicide Event Report
DONSIR	Department of the Navy Suicide Incident Report
DOTMLPF	doctrine, organization, training, materiel, leadership, personnel, and facilities
EMS	emergency medical services
EMT	emergency medical technician
ESAP	Expeditionary Substance Abuse Program
ESB	Executive Safety Board
Ex	echelon (where x = echelon number; e.g., E1)
EXORD	executive order
FFSC	Fleet and Family Support Center
FST	Frontline Supervisors Training
FTE	full-time equivalent

FY	fiscal year
G-1	Deputy Chief of Staff for Army Personnel
G-3	Deputy Chief of Staff for Army Operations
GMT	General Military Training
HQMC	Marine Corps Headquarters
HSS	Health Service Support
IDS	Integrated Delivery System
IED	improvised explosive device
IOM	Institute of Medicine
IPT	Integrated Product Team
IRB	Investment Review Board
ISRT	Installation Suicide Response Team
ITS	Individual Training Standard
LINK	look for possible concerns, inquire about concerns, note level of risk, and know referral sources and strategies
LIS	local implementation study
LPSP	Limited Privilege Suicide Prevention
MAJCOM	major command
MARADMIN	Marine Corps administrative memorandum
MCCS	Marine Corps Community Services
MCMAP	Marine Corps Martial Arts Program
MCO	Marine Corps order
MCRP	Marine Corps reference publication
MCSPP	Marine Corps Suicide Prevention Program
MEDCOM	U.S. Army Medical Command
MEPRS	Medical Expense and Performance Reporting System
MHAT	Mental Health Advisory Team
MNF-I	Multi-National Force—Iraq

MOS	military occupational specialty
MOSST	Marine Corps Operational Stress Surveillance and Training
MTF	medical treatment facility
MWR	Family and Morale, Welfare and Recreation Command
NAMI	National Alliance on Mental Illness
NAVADMIN	Navy administrative memorandum
NAVPERS	Navy Personnel Command
NCO	noncommissioned officer
NDRI	National Defense Research Institute
NETC	Naval Education and Training Command
NG	National Guard
NGB/CF	Director of the Air National Guard
NIMH	National Institute of Mental Health
NKO	Navy Knowledge Online
NMCPHC	Navy and Marine Corps Public Health Center
NOSC	Naval Operational Support Center
NQMP	National Quality Management Program
NREPP	National Registry of Evidence-Based Programs and Practices
NSPL	National Suicide Prevention Lifeline
OAFME	Office of the Armed Forces Medical Examiner
OEF	Operation Enduring Freedom
OIF	Operation Iraqi Freedom
OPNAV N135	Personal Readiness and Community Support Branch
OPNAVINST	Office of the Chief of Naval Operations instruction
OSC	Operational Stress Control
OSCAR	Operational Stress Control and Readiness
OTSG	Office of the Surgeon General

PAM	pamphlet
PCR	Personnel Casualty Report
PDHA	Post-Deployment Health Assessment
PDHRA	Post-Deployment Health Reassessment
PDRL	permanent disability retired list
PH	psychological health
PITE	Point-in-Time Extract
POC	point of contact
POD	plan of the day
PRESS	prepare, recognize, engage, send, sustain
PSA	public service announcement
PTSD	posttraumatic stress disorder
QI	quality improvement
QPR	question, persuade, refer
RACE	Recognize changes in your marine; ask your marine directly whether he or she is thinking about killing him- or herself; care for your marine by calmly controlling the situation, listening without judgment, and removing any means that the marine could use to inflict self-injury; and escort your marine to the chain of command, a chaplain, mental health professional, or primary-care provider.
RC	Reserve Component
RESPECT-Mil	Re-Engineering Systems of Primary Care Treatment in the Military
RRP	Risk Reduction Program
RTD	return to duty
RWW	Returning Warriors Workshop
SAF/FMB	Secretary of the Air Force for Budget
SAF/MRM	Secretary of the Air Force for Force Management Integration
SAF/PA	Secretary of the Air Force for Public Affairs

SAMHSA	Substance Abuse and Mental Health Services Administration
SBIRT	Screening, Brief Intervention, and Referral to Treatment
SESS	Suicide Event Surveillance System
SMS	short message service
SOAR	Suicide, Options, Awareness, and Relief
SOS	Signs of Suicide
SPAN	Suicide Prevention Action Network
SPARRC	Suicide Prevention and Risk Reduction Committee
SPC	suicide-prevention coordinator
SPO	suicide program officer
SPPM	suicide-prevention program manager
SPRC	Suicide Prevention Resource Center
SPRINT	Special Psychiatric Rapid Intervention Team
SRMSO	Suicide Risk Management and Surveillance Office
SRT	Suicide Response Team
SSRI	selective serotonin-reuptake inhibitor
T2	National Center for Telehealth and Technology
TBI	traumatic brain injury
TDRL	temporary disability retired list
TECOM	Training and Education Command
TRADOC	U.S. Army Training and Doctrine Command
TSP	training support package
TSR	traumatic stress response
UCMJ	Uniform Code of Military Justice
USAF	U.S. Air Force
USMC	U.S. Marine Corps
VA	U.S. Department of Veterans Affairs

VEILS   Virtual Experience Immersive Learning Simulation

VHA   Veterans Health Administration

WAQ   Warrior Adventure Quest

WRAIR   Walter Reed Army Institute of Research

CHAPTER ONE

Introduction

Background

As the United States enters its ninth year of continuous combat in Afghanistan and Iraq, concerns about the stresses on U.S. forces generated by repetitive deployments to war zones have been heightened. All services have experienced increases in suicides, especially the Army and Marine Corps, whose forces have borne the brunt of combat in these theaters. The Army appears poised to have a record number of suicides in 2009 relative to the recent past.[1]

Today, the U.S. Department of Defense (DoD) remains actively engaged in efforts to prevent suicide. Each service employs a myriad of specific prevention campaigns. A DoD-wide committee with representation from each service and other relevant agencies meets monthly to share information. Each year, there is a DoD-sponsored conference on suicide prevention (now cosponsored by the U.S. Department of Veterans Affairs [VA]) attended by a range of DoD representatives, including behavioral health-care providers and chaplains.

Study Purpose

The recent increase in suicides across the services prompted leaders to ask, "What more can be done to prevent suicides among servicemembers?" This study represents a first step in responding to this question. This study focused on four objectives:

- Review the current evidence detailing suicide epidemiology in the military.
- Identify state-of-the-art suicide-prevention programs.
- Describe and catalog suicide-prevention activities in DoD and across each service.
- Recommend ways to ensure that the activities in DoD and across each service reflect best practices.

---

[1] As of November 16, 2009, the Army reported 140 active-duty suicides, which is equivalent to the total in 2008. It also reported 71 suicides by soldiers not on active duty, more than its total in 2008 (DoD, 2009b).

DoD is expressly concerned with an increase in suicide deaths; consequently, our monograph focuses predominantly on this outcome. When relevant, however, we provide some information on nonfatal suicidal behaviors, including suicide attempts and thoughts of killing oneself (i.e., suicide ideation). We present some information on the epidemiology of such behaviors among military personnel (Chapter Two), as well as highlight when such outcomes are used to evaluate suicide-prevention programs (Chapter Three).

Approach

Information about suicide among military personnel and the programs aimed at preventing suicide is not located in one place. As we detail in this monograph, different organizations and agencies are responsible for preventing suicides across DoD. As a result, our research involved outreach to many of these organizations. We identified and read all policy statements on suicide prevention and any available description about existing programs. We also attended the 2009 DoD/VA Suicide Prevention Conference. We conducted key informant interviews with persons knowledgeable about suicide prevention in DoD and across each service. Interviews were conducted with persons or representatives from organizations responsible for generating or delivering suicide-prevention programs and initiatives. Those willing to be interviewed provided names of potential key informants, and we continued to conduct interviews until we determined that we were not learning additional information. Key informants provided descriptions of programs and initiatives, including the intent of each specific initiative, its history, its source of funding, and plans for its sustainability. We synthesized the information gleaned from the literature and from interviews across five domains, described in Chapters Four and Five. In Table 1.1, we present the individuals with whom we spoke who agreed to have their names listed in this monograph.

To identify best practices in preventing suicide, we reviewed the literature, specifically targeting empirical and review papers. We focused on larger syntheses of the literature that are guiding current work in suicide prevention nationally (Goldsmith et al., 2002), an unpublished synthesis of the literature produced by the National Institute of Mental Health (NIMH) on behalf of the Department of the Army (Schoenbaum, Heinssen, and Pearson, 2009), and the final report of the Blue Ribbon Work Group on Suicide Prevention in the Veteran Population (2008). We attended the 2009 annual meeting of the American Association of Suicidology (AAS). We also interviewed 13 experts who demonstrated a strong record of publications on suicide in peer-reviewed scientific journals. Interviews lasted about one hour and focused on the following topics:

- evaluation methods for suicide-prevention practices

Table 1.1
Key Informant Interviewees in the U.S. Department of Defense

Interviewee	Affiliation
Sandra Black	CHPPM[a]
James Cartwright	CHPPM
LCDR Bonnie Chavez	SPPM, U.S. Navy
CAPT Jonathan Frusti	Armed Forces Chaplain Board
Margaret Kibben	Navy Chaplain Corps
Lt. Col. Michael Kindt	SPPM, U.S. Air Force
CPT L. Languirand	U.S. Army
Mark Long	NMCPHC
BG Colleen McGuire	U.S. Army
John Reibling	SPPM, U.S. Coast Guard
Kathy Robertson	Navy Youth Program
CAPT Virginia Torsch	Navy Reserve Psychological Health Outreach Program
LTC Scott Weichl	CHPPM
LCDR Aaron Werbel	SPPM, U.S. Marine Corps

NOTE: CHPPM = U.S. Army Center for Health Promotion and Preventive Medicine. SPPM = suicide-prevention program manager. NMCPHC = Navy and Marine Corps Public Health Center.

[a] CHPPM is in the process of changing to the U.S. Army Public Health Command (see APHC, 2010).

- descriptions of programs that have been rigorously evaluated
- what the research suggests are the most-effective suicide-prevention programs across the spectrum of primary prevention to postvention (defined in more detail in Chapter Three)
- programs that hold the most promise for preventing suicide in DoD
- practices that would or would not be recommended for preventing suicide in DoD.

The information gathered from our literature review and from our expert interviews was used to evaluate the effectiveness of different suicide-prevention initiatives, with specific attention to their applicability in the military environment (described in Chapter Three). In Table 1.2, we present the individuals with whom we spoke who agreed to have their names listed in this monograph.

All research was conducted between September 2008 and November 2009. All key informant interviews were conducted by telephone or in person and began with

Table 1.2
Key Informant Interviewees Outside the U.S. Department of Defense

Interviewee	Affiliation
Brian Altman	SPAN USA
Gregory K. Brown	University of Pennsylvania
Martha Bruce	Weill Cornell Medical College
COL Charles Engel	Uniformed Services University of the Health Sciences
Marjan Holloway	Uniformed Services University of the Health Sciences
David Jobes	Catholic University of America
Thomas Joiner	University of Florida
Marsha Linehan	University of Washington
David Litts	SPRC
John Mann	Columbia University
Ken Norton	NAMI New Hampshire
Jane Pearson	NIMH
Michael Schoenbaum	NIMH

NOTE: SPAN = Suicide Prevention Action Network. SPRC = Suicide Prevention Resource Center. NAMI = National Alliance on Mental Illness.

a description of the study and spoken consent to participate. All procedures were reviewed and approved by the RAND Human Subjects Protection Committee and had DoD second-level Investment Review Board (IRB) approval.

Organization of This Monograph

This report has six chapters. Chapter Two provides information on the epidemiology of suicide. We organize this information according to quantity (number and rate of suicides in the military and relative to the general population), the location of suicides across demographic and military characteristics, and the causes and correlates of suicide, and conclude with a discussion of the mechanisms proposed to explain why people take their own lives. Chapter Three reviews the scientific evidence bearing on suicide prevention across two domains: prevention programs designed for all individuals and those targeted to individuals who are uniquely at risk of harming themselves. In both of these chapters, we highlight why findings from the scientific literature have specific relevance to the military. Chapter Four is divided into four sections that represent each of the four services studied (Army, Navy, Air Force, Marine Corps). We provide a description of the philosophy guiding suicide prevention in each service and an overview of prevention activities for each service. Chapter Five, also divided into four sections that represent each of the four services, describes how suicide-prevention programs are supported with respect to official documentation bearing on suicide, organizations responsible for preventing suicide, and funding for suicide prevention. The monograph concludes with Chapter Six, which summarizes the degree to which the services' prevention programs represent state-of-the-art practices and provides recommendations on how DoD suicide-prevention activities could be enhanced to be comprehensive and reflect state-of-the-art practice. In appendixes, we provide a compendium with detailed information on each unique suicide-prevention initiative in each of the four services. These appendixes were vetted for accuracy and comprehensiveness by the Navy, Marine Corps, and Air Force SPPMs and staff of the Army Suicide Prevention Task Force (ASPTF).

CHAPTER TWO

The Epidemiology of Suicide in the Military

This chapter presents the most-currently available data on suicide in the U.S. military, along with a discussion of the research challenges particular to epidemiologic investigations of suicide. We did not set out to be comprehensive in our review of the epidemiologic literature on suicide. Rather, we intended only to highlight research findings that we considered relevant to DoD. This chapter deals with such questions of interest to policymakers as what the suicide rate is in the services, whether it differs from that of a comparable segment of the civilian population, how it has changed over time, how it varies between and within the military services, and who is most at risk. Throughout, we place information seen as most pertinent to the military in text boxes to highlight those points.

This chapter presents information in four of the five sections that correspond with four of the five rubrics of epidemiology: quantity, location and variation, causes, and mechanism (Anthony and Van Etten, 1998). The section on *quantity* deals with the number of U.S. servicemembers who die by suicide, along with information about how the rate in DoD and in each service compares with the suicide rate in the general population of the United States. The section on *location and variation* provides evidence about how death by suicide among servicemembers varies across demographic characteristics (gender, age, race and ethnicity), geography, over time, and across military-specific factors (i.e., rank, component, and deployment). Discussion of *causes* of suicide reviews relevant correlates and risk factors for suicide: Which factors are associated with suicide among military personnel, and, if possible to determine, which factors increase servicemembers' risk of dying by suicide? A section on *mechanism* draws on psychological theory to review the conditions that have been hypothesized to lead to an individual's decision to take his or her own life. There is a fifth rubric, prevention and control, and we devote Chapter Three entirely to this important domain.

Quantity: The Number of U.S. Servicemembers Who Die by Suicide

What Is Suicide?

When analyzing suicides, words and definitions matter. Tracking suicides using a clearly defined nomenclature helps ensure identification of valid trends over time and across populations. For this reason, defining terms is typically the first step in prevention efforts and provides data with which prevention and intervention efforts can be evaluated and accurately target groups at highest risk. The range of behaviors that fall under the umbrella of self-directed violence is wide, and researchers and organizations have disagreed about the terms and definitions that should be used to describe them. The Centers for Disease Control and Prevention (CDC) is currently devising a national suicide nomenclature to ensure consistent terminology in reporting on suicide and related behaviors to improve communication, research, and prevention efforts, though it had not been published at the time of this writing (Crosby and Ortega, 2009). In 2009, a DoD/VA working group on suicide nomenclature was convened to standardize suicide nomenclature across the two agencies. The working group has agreed to adopt the CDC nomenclature when it is released. In addition, in calendar year (CY) 2008, all services adopted the Department of Defense Suicide Event Report (DoDSER) to track data on completed suicides and some suicide attempts in the services, though, as of this writing, the summary report for CY 2008 had not yet been released.

A number of different definitions of *suicide* exist across the literature (i.e., De Leo et al., 2006; O'Carroll, Berman, et al., 1996; Posner et al., 2007; Silverman et al., 2007), though all generally refer to suicide as a *self-inflicted behavior that results in a fatal injury and for which there is evidence of some intent to die as a result of the behavior* (Posner et al., 2007). Additionally, a range of suicidal behaviors exist that may include thoughts of harming or killing oneself (i.e., suicide ideation), writing a suicide note, making an attempt that does not result in death, overdosing on drugs that a person knows might kill him or her, and making an attempt that is interrupted before a person dies.

Implications for DoD

Standardizing nomenclature and data collection within DoD and the VA is an important step in preventing suicide in both organizations and will help ensure accurate communication both within and between these organizations.

Tracking Suicides. The Office of the Armed Forces Medical Examiner (OAFME) determines the cause of death for all active-duty deaths, which includes deaths among members of the active component and activated reservists and members of the National Guard (NG) (Pearse, undated). At a meeting of the DoD Suicide Prevention and Risk

Reduction Committee (SPARRC) on October 27, 2008, we were informed of the process by which the OAFME makes such determinations, and OAFME staff provided further elaboration. Cause of death is determined by OAFME medical examiners for deaths over which that office has jurisdiction. The OAFME also reviews civilian autopsies for suspect deaths outside of its jurisdiction to validate suicide cases. The OAFME follows national medical-examiner guidelines for identifying suicide cases and, for self-inflicted firearm fatalities, determines a death to be a suicide if there is evidence that the victim intentionally pulled the trigger.

As of 2006, a DoD working group under the direction of Health Affairs required that, when producing estimates of suicides, all services include in their counts of "active-duty suicides" the following five categories:

1.   all regular-component servicemembers except deserters (including personnel on appellate leave)
2.   reserve commissioned officers and cadets and midshipmen at service academies
3.   regular-component personnel whose suicide-related death occurred while on the temporary or permanent disability retired list (TDRL/PDRL) for 120 days or less (including those on TDRL while comatose from a suicide attempt)
4.   all active NG reserve (full-time support personnel) and activated Guard and reservists
5.   all Guard and reserve members who die by suicide en route to or during (a) initial active-duty training (boot camp and entry-level training), (b) two-week annual training, or (c) weekend inactive-duty training.

This process therefore excludes any suicides among reservists not on active duty. In April 2009, Senators Lindsey Graham and Ben Nelson instructed each service to develop a plan to track suicides among members of the Reserve Component (RC) and NG not on active duty. The Under Secretary of Defense for Personnel and Readiness has implemented a plan to report suicides that occur on or after January 1, 2009 (Embrey, 2009b). Specifically, each service is responsible for reporting suicide data among Selected Reserve members not activated, mobilized, or in training that will be forwarded to the OAFME. To date, there is no requirement or plan for the OAFME to validate suicide cases identified among nonactivated reservists where cause of death is determined outside of the OAFME.

Table 2.1
Suicide Count and Rate per 100,000 in the Department of Defense and for Each Service, 2001–2008

Year	DoD N	DoD Rate	Army N	Army Rate	Navy N	Navy Rate	Air Force N	Air Force Rate	Marines N	Marines Rate
2001– 2008	1,609	12.1	712	13.1	325	10.5	331	10.3	241	15.4
2001– 2006	1,117	11.2	457	11.6	244	10.2	250	10.1	166	14.6
2001	160	10.3	52	9.0	40	10.0	38	9.7	30	16.7
2002	171	10.3	70	11.5	45	10.9	33	7.4	23	12.5
2003	190	11.0	79	11.4	44	10.8	41	9.6	26	13.4
2004	194	11.3	67	9.6	40	10.0	53	12.6	34	17.5
2005	189	11.3	87	12.7	37	9.5	37	9.3	28	14.4
2006	213	13.1	102	15.3	38	10.1	48	12.2	25	12.9
2007	224	13.8	115	16.7	40	11.1	36	9.5	33	16.5
2008	268	16.3	139	19.3	41	11.7	46	12.6	42	19.9

SOURCE: Mortality Surveillance Division, Armed Forces Medical Examiner (as of April 1, 2010).

Implications for DoD

Current estimates of suicide counts and rates in DoD exclude non-activated reservists. Efforts to include nonactivated reservists are planned but will be challenging, as there is known variation in cause-of-death determinations outside the OAFME and no plans yet within the OAFME to validate these cases (see "Comparison with the U.S. Adult Population" later in this chapter).

Recent Estimates

Each service has an SPPM responsible for presenting to that service's leadership updated suicide statistics. The most-recent estimates of the number of confirmed suicides across DoD and for each service specifically, are presented in Table 2.1.

Calculating the Department of Defense Suicide Rate

A rate is an estimate of the frequency of an event relative to a unit of time. Thus, the rates presented in Table 2.1 represent the frequency of suicides for the population at risk over a one-year interval (except for the first two rows, which present the rate from

Table 2.2
Suicides in the United States, by Year

Year	N	Rate per 100,000
2001	30,622	10.74
2002	31,655	11.00
2003	31,484	10.84
2004	32,439	11.06
2005	32,637	11.03
2006	33,300	11.15

2001 to 2008 and 2001 to 2006). In DoD and in the United States more generally, suicide is a rare event, with one case per every 10,000 people (see Table 2.2). Thus, for ease of interpretation, suicide rates are typically presented per 100,000 population.

The denominator used to estimate the suicide rate is intended to represent those individuals at risk for being in the numerator (i.e., suicide cases) over the course of the specific year and thus must reflect the five groups identified earlier. This number changes on a daily basis, so assumptions must be made about how to approximate the denominator. In 2006, the DoD Suicide Rate Standardization Work Group determined that the denominator would reflect two components that comprise the "total force" of a given calendar year: the active component and reserve full-time equivalent (FTE). The workgroup determined that the estimated size of the active component be the recorded September end-strengths of the active component in a given calendar year. To estimate reserve FTE, workgroup members devised the following formula:

$$\text{Reserve FTE} = \big[(\text{Selected Reserve} - \text{AGR} - \text{CTS}) \times 11\%\big] + \text{AGR} + \text{CTS}, \quad (2.1)$$

where AGR = Active Guard and Reserve and CTS = called to serve.

Here, Selected Reserve consists of those who attended annual training for two weeks, those who attended inactive-duty training over the course of a weekend, and those who participated in initial active-duty training (i.e., reserve basic training). Excluding those who met criteria for both Selected Reserve and either AGR (reservists employed full time in units and organizations that support the RC) or those who have been activated (CTS), the workgroup determined that each member of the remaining group spent approximately 11 percent of the year at risk of being in the numerator. This value is represented in square brackets. All AGR and CTS personnel are assumed to be at risk for the entire calendar year.

Variability in Rate Estimates

A sampling error is associated with the published suicide rate for each service and across DoD. Acknowledging this variability is particularly important when examining trends over time. We found no published estimate of the error associated with the estimated suicide rate for DoD or for each service, so we calculated our own. From the published number of suicide cases in a given year and the corresponding rate, we were able to calculate the denominator used for each estimate using the following formula:

$$\text{Denominator} = \frac{\text{number of suicide cases} \times 100,000}{\text{rate per } 100,000}. \tag{2.2}$$

Using the denominator we derived in Equation 2.2, we calculated approximate 95-percent confidence intervals using the normal approximation to the binomial distribution:

$$\text{Rate} \pm 1.96 \times \sqrt{\frac{\text{rate}(1 - \text{rate})}{\text{denominator}}}. \tag{2.3}$$

The 95-percent confidence intervals indicate the reliability of the calculated suicide rate. They represent the range in which the estimated suicide rate would fall 95 percent of the time if calculated on repeated samples. The evidence suggests that rates differ significantly over time when there is no overlap in the corresponding confidence intervals. The results from our calculations are discussed and illustrated in the section "Temporal Trends" later in this chapter.

Implications for DoD

We found no published DoD document that presented estimates of the sampling error associated with published suicide rates. Ignoring this error makes comparing rates over time almost impossible.

Comparison with the U.S. Adult Population

Producing National Suicide Estimates. National data on suicides are derived from local death-certificate registries forwarded by states to the National Center for Health Statistics at the CDC. The CDC (2006) reports that it releases injury mortality statistics approximately 18 months after a year's end. However, as of this writing (October 2009), the most-recent national data available were for CY 2006. The delay in reporting is due to procedural issues involved in collecting, compiling, verifying, and preparing these data.

Verification of suicide data is particularly important, because there is known variation in suicide statistics across four domains. First, there is no standardized way in which suicides are defined or how ambiguous cases (e.g., Russian-roulette deaths) are classified across the country. Second, there are differences across states in the prerequisite qualifications for professionals charged by law with certifying a death as a suicide (offices of coroner and medical examiner) (Hanzlick, 1996). Third, there are differences in the extent to which possible suicide cases are investigated. Lastly, regions and states differ in the quality of their data management (Goldsmith et al., 2002).

Acknowledging these data limitations, we find that the number of suicides has hovered around 30,000 per year in the United States between 1999 and 2006 (range: 29,199 in 1999 to 33,300 in 2006). This translates to an average crude suicide rate of 10.84 per 100,000 persons (range: 10.43 in 2000 to 11.15 in 2006). The estimated annual suicide rate in the general population, presented for years from 2001 to 2006 in Table 2.2, hovers at around 0.01 percent or 10 per 100,000 (CDC, 2010).

Comparison with DoD and Each Service. The lag in release of national data makes it impossible to make timely comparisons between the military suicide rate and the population at large. As of this writing, we could compare rates only from the most recent year for which we have national data, 2006.

Comparing the crude U.S. rate with DoD-wide and service-specific rates indicates that the suicide rate is higher in DoD and in each service of the military than the general population. However, military personnel included in the DoD suicide rate differ from the general population in important ways that affect the estimated suicide rate. We discuss many of these differences in this chapter in our section on variation. Of note, the age, sex, and racial composition of active-duty military personnel differs from that of the general population, and (as discussed later), suicide is known to vary across these domains.

Thus, when comparing rates between DoD and the U.S. general population, it is important to adjust for known differences between the groups. Although such adjustments have been made by DoD and by each service, their methods are not transparent. Thus, we performed our own calculations. We used direct adjustment to calculate an adjusted national suicide rate for a synthetic national population having the same demographic profile of DoD personnel and of each service. To do this, we calculated the number of military personnel in one of 240 sex × age × race × ethnicity strata for years 2001–2006 using the Defense Enrollment Eligibility Reporting System (DEERS) Point-in-Time Extract (PITE) provided by the Defense Manpower Data Center (DMDC). The DEERS PITE contains monthly extracts of demographic data for all servicemembers (active duty and reservists serving more than 30 days) who are eligible for medical benefits, and thus represents a complete monthly snapshot of U.S. military personnel. A total count was calculated by extracting personnel data from

September of each year on the individual's service, component, race, ethnicity, sex, and age. Weighted tabulations were produced by year for sex, race or ethnic category, age group, and service using a weighting scheme designed to replicate the denominator used by DoD. A weight of 1 was assigned to all active-duty personnel and AGR, and a weight of 0.11 was assigned to non-AGR reservists. We estimated the crude U.S. suicide rate for each of the 240 strata. We then multiplied the stratum-specific suicide rate to the number of military personnel within each stratum to estimate the number of expected suicides per stratum. We added the total number of expected suicides and divided by the total population to arrive at a nationally adjusted suicide rate. Comparisons between the military suicide rate and the adjusted national rate are provided in Table 2.3.

The estimates presented in Table 2.3 show that, between 2001 and 2004, the DoD suicide rate was a little more than half of what one would expect given the demographic profile of DoD. However, in recent years, the DoD rate has risen while the U.S. rate has remained relatively constant, thereby narrowing the gap between the two (we discuss temporal trends in more detail later in this chapter). Furthermore, if one assumes the national rate to remain constant in 2007 and 2008, the gap between the DoD rate and the national rate may become even narrower. We also created an adjusted national rate for each service and compared this with each service's actual rate. That is, we calculated what we would expect the U.S. Marine Corps (USMC) rate to be by adjusting the national statistics to reflect the age-sex-race-ethnicity profile of USMC. Looking specifically at the rate within each service, the same relationship seen for DoD is apparent for the Army and Navy, though there is no evidence that the gap between the Navy's suicide rate and that of the general population narrowed in 2006 as it did for the Army and for DoD as a whole. Across services, USMC has generally the highest estimated suicide rate. In 2002, the expected rate was 19.7, and the actual rate was 12.5, which is 63 percent of 19.7. In 2004, the expected rate was 19.5, and the actual rate was 17.5, which is 90 percent of 19.5. The relationship between the Air Force suicide rate and the adjusted national rate fluctuates over time and was as low as 39 percent of the expected rate in 2002, though it was as high as 66 percent in 2004.

Table 2.3
Department of Defense and Service-Specific Suicide Rates and U.S. Rate Adjusted by Service

Year	DoD			Army			Navy			Air Force			Marines		
	N	Rate	U.S. Adjusted Rate	N	Rate	U.S. Adjusted Rate	N	Rate	U.S. Adjusted Rate	N	Rate	U.S. Adjusted Rate	N	Rate	U.S. Adjusted Rate
2001–2008	1,609	12.2	N/A	711	13.2	N/A	325	10.5	N/A	332	10.4	N/A	241	15.5	N/A
2001–2006	1,117	11.2	19.1	457	11.6	18.8	244	10.2	19.9	250	10.1	19.0	166	14.6	19.5
2001	160	10.3	19.1	52	9.0	18.7	40	10.0	20.2	38	9.7	18.8	30	16.7	19.6
2002	171	10.3	19.3	70	11.5	18.9	45	10.9	20.2	33	7.4	19.1	23	12.5	19.7
2003	190	11.0	19.0	79	11.4	18.7	44	10.8	19.7	41	9.6	18.9	26	13.4	19.3
2004	194	11.3	19.2	67	9.6	18.9	40	10.0	19.9	53	12.6	19.1	34	17.5	19.5
2005	189	11.3	18.9	87	12.7	18.4	37	9.5	19.4	37	9.3	19.0	28	14.4	19.3
2006	213	13.1	19.2	102	15.3	18.9	38	10.1	19.8	48	12.2	19.0	25	12.9	19.6
2007	224	13.8	N/A	115	16.7	N/A	40	11.1	N/A	36	9.5	N/A	33	16.5	N/A
2008	268	16.3	N/A	139	19.3	N/A	41	11.7	N/A	46	12.6	N/A	42	19.9	N/A

SOURCE: DoD data from Mortality Surveillance Division, Armed Forces Medical Examiner (as of April 1, 2010).

NOTE: N/A = not applicable.

> ## Implications for DoD
>
> Due to prompt reporting of suicides among military personnel and lagged reporting among the general population, temporal trends may appear among military personnel before they are observed among the general U.S. population.
>
> Lagged national data make it impossible to make timely comparisons between the military population and the national average.
>
> The suicide rate in the military has historically been lower than the adjusted national rate. However, the gap between the rates is narrowing, primarily in the Army.

Suicide Attempts

Suicides are suicide attempts resulting in fatal injury, though a larger number of individuals who attempt suicide are either not fatally injured or not injured at all. Two methods are used to track suicide attempts: individuals' self-report of having had previously attempted suicide, and events classified by a third party as being a suicide attempt. Both methods have strengths and limitations. Self-reports of suicide attempts tend to rely on respondents providing their own interpretation of what constitutes an attempt, which, without clarification, may overestimate prevalence because respondents may consider ideas or behaviors to be attempts that are not typically classified as such, such as thoughts about suicide or making a plan to kill oneself (Meehan et al., 1992). On the other hand, third-party reports rely primarily on information from clinical settings, such as emergency rooms, that may underestimate actual prevalence because they tend to capture only the most-severe suicidal behaviors (Birkhead et al., 1993).

Self-Report of Suicide Attempts. Active-duty military personnel are asked about past suicide attempts in the DoD Survey of Health Related Behaviors Among Active Duty Military Personnel. Data from the 2008 survey indicate that close to 6 percent of active-duty military personnel have attempted suicide in the past: Approximately 3 percent reported having attempted suicide since joining the military (2.1 percent in the past year and 1.1 percent since joining the military but not in the past year) and 2.5 percent reported having attempted suicide before joining the military but not in the past year (Bray, Pemberton, et al., 2009). These rates can be compared to a nationally representative 2008 survey of U.S. household members, which found that 0.5 percent of adults (ages 18 and older) made a suicide attempt in the past year (SAMHSA, 2009). For the first time, in 2006, a health behavior survey was conducted among a sample of the Guard/RC of the military, though, at the time of this writing, the results had not yet been released (RTI International, 2008).

Third-Party Reports of Suicide Attempts. In 2004, the Army established the Army Medical Department (AMEDD) Suicide Risk Management and Surveillance Office (SRMSO). SRMSO developed a webform called the Army Suicide Event Report (ASER) that a credentialed behavioral health provider at each medical treatment facility (MTF) was required to complete for any event in which an active-duty Army soldier died by suicide or was hospitalized or evacuated for a suicide attempt. In 2006, 896 ASERs were completed for suicide attempts (SRMSO, 2007). In CY 2007, there were 935 ASERs submitted for suicide attempts, categorized according to a definition by the World Health Organization to include "any act with a non-fatal outcome, in which an individual deliberately initiates a non-habitual behavior that, without intervention from others, will cause self-harm" (Platt et al., 1992). We found no published data on suicide attempts in the Navy, Air Force, or Marine Corps, though all services will be presenting such data for CY 2008 as part of the DoDSER program.

In the general population, between 2001 and 2007, hospital emergency departments saw between 323,370 (in 2001) and 425,650 (in 2004) cases of confirmed or suspected self-inflicted nonfatal injuries, with crude rates ranging from 112.9 per 100,000 in 2002 to 145.3 per 100,000 in 2004, indicating roughly ten to 14 attempts for every suicide death (CDC, 2010). In 2005, there were 202,700 inpatient hospitalizations in the United States resulting from self-inflicted violence, which may have occurred with or without suicidal intent. Just over 1 percent of these individuals died in the hospital. Hospitalizations resulting from self-inflicted violence lasted an average of four days and cost in total approximately $1.1 billion (Russo, Owens, and Hambrick, 2008).

Implications for DoD

Most recent evidence suggests that approximately 3 percent of members of the active component had attempted to kill themselves since joining the military. This is likely an overestimate and may include suicidal behaviors not typically classified as attempts.

Beginning in 2008, the services adopted a common surveillance system called DoDSER, which was developed by a workgroup consisting of representatives from each service. Since it relies on third-party reports of attempts, DoDSER will underestimate the actual prevalence of suicide attempts and reflect only the most severe (i.e., those that resulted in emergency medical care).

Suicide Ideation

Suicide ideation refers to a range of thinking, from passive thoughts of wanting to be dead to active thoughts of harming or killing oneself (Goldsmith et al., 2002; Posner et al., 2007). Many more people think about killing themselves than actually do: Compared to a national suicide rate of 0.01 percent, 3.7 percent of adults in the United States in 2008 reported serious thoughts about killing themselves in the past year (SAMHSA, 2009). Individuals' self-reports are the primary source of information on suicide ideation, though some people will present to third parties, such as emergency departments, having thought about taking their own lives though not having engaged in self-injurious behavior.

In 2008, close to 12 percent of active-duty military personnel reported having seriously considered suicide in the past: 4.6 percent in the past year, 3.3 percent since joining the service but not in the past year, and 3.8 percent seriously considered suicide prior to joining the military but not in the past year (Bray, Pemberton, et al., 2009). Estimates of suicide ideation are also collected among military personnel returning from deployments. One month after the ground war began in Iraq in 2003, service-members returning from deployments (mostly from Iraq and Afghanistan in support of Operation Iraqi Freedom [OIF] and Operation Enduring Freedom [OEF]) have been required to complete the Post-Deployment Health Assessment (PDHA) (Hoge, Auchterlonie, and Milliken, 2006). The instrument asks, "during the last 2 weeks, how often have you been bothered by . . . thoughts that you would be better off dead or hurting yourself in some way?" (DoD, 2008). Among soldiers and marines who completed the assessment between May 1, 2003, and April 30, 2004, 1.3 percent of OIF veterans, 0.8 percent of OEF veterans, and 0.7 percent of those returning from deployments in other locations reported having some or many such thoughts (Hoge, Auchterlonie, and Milliken, 2006).

Suicide ideation among soldiers resulting in hospitalization or evacuation is captured on the ASER. In 2006, there were 52 ASERs completed for hospitalizations or evacuations resulting from suicide ideation only (i.e., no self-harm). However, in 2006, not all Army medical facilities were aware that noninjurious suicidal behaviors warranted an ASER. When AMEDD clarified in 2007 that ASERs were to be completed for hospitalizations and evacuations resulting from ideation only, the estimated number of third-party reports of ideation alone (i.e., no self-harm) increased dramatically to 622.

Implications for DoD

In 2008, approximately one in ten active-component servicemembers reported thoughts about killing themselves since joining the military. Many fewer will actually die by suicide, but this prevalence highlights the need to increase awareness and foster communication about suicide and suicide prevention in the military.

Variation: Where Suicides Are Located in the U.S. Military

The second rubric of epidemiology, *location or variation*, describes where suicides exist. We provide this information for the country as a whole and for the military specifically across four domains: demographic characteristics, geography, time, and military-specific characteristics.

Demographics

When comparing rates of suicide in the military with those of the U.S. population, we controlled for differences between the two groups with respect to gender, age, and race and ethnicity (see Table 2.3). We did this because there are known differences in rates of suicide across these categories, which we describe in this section.

Gender Differences. In the United States, approximately 80 to 85 percent of all military personnel are male, compared with roughly half of the U.S. civilian population (U.S. Census Bureau, 2010; DoD, undated). In the United States, as is the case in most countries across the world, males are more likely than females to die by suicide (Goldsmith et al., 2002), though females are more likely to make suicide attempts (Hawton, 2000). The most probable explanation for this is that men who try to kill themselves tend to use more lethal means, such as firearms, while women use more reversible methods, such as overdose (Goldsmith et al., 2002; Mann, 2002).

Similar trends are seen in each military service, where suicides disproportionately occur among male servicemembers. Of all suicides between 1999 and 2007, the suicide rate for men in the Navy was 11.9 per 100,000, and, in the Marine Corps, it was 15.2 per 100,000, compared with a rate among women that was 3.6 and 4.8 per 100,000 for the Navy and Marine Corps, respectively (Hilton et al., 2009). In CY 2006, the rate for male soldiers was close to twice what it was for female soldiers: 17.82 versus 11.33 per 100,000. In CY 2007, females accounted for 5 percent of all suicides, though they comprised 14 percent of the total Army force (SRMSO, 2007, 2008). In CY 2007, 100 percent of suicide victims in the Air Force were male (Loftus, 2008b).

Age Differences. In general, the rate of suicide increases as a function of age, increasing sharply during adolescence to a point at which the rate reaches a plateau and stays more or less constant until the later years of life, when it increases dramatically for men (though it decreases for women) (CDC, 2010; McKeown, Cuffe, and Schulz, 2006). In Figures 2.1 and 2.2, we present the number of suicides in the general population and the corresponding rate, respectively, for CY 2006 as a function of sex and age.

In aggregate, the age distribution for military personnel skews younger than the age distribution of civilian adults in the United States: Almost half of active-duty personnel and one-third of selected reservists are between 18 and 25 (DoD, undated). For sailors and marines, there are not large differences in rates of suicide across age categories, though one could conclude that the rate for older sailors and marines tends to be a bit higher. For example, between 1999 and 2007, the suicide rate in the Navy was

Figure 2.1
Suicides, by Age, in the United States, Calendar Year 2006

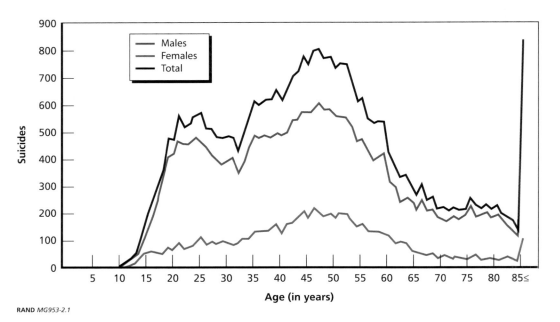

RAND *MG953-2.1*

Figure 2.2
Suicides, by Age, in the United States, Rate per 100,000, Calendar Year 2006

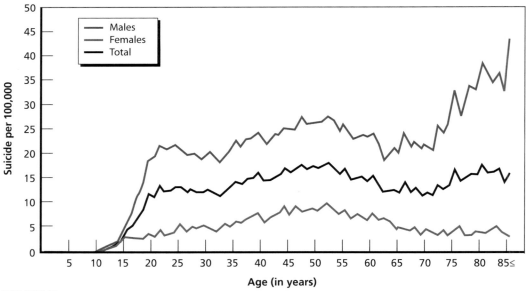

RAND *MG953-2.2*

approximately 13.7 per 100,000 among those 45–54, while it was between 10 and 11 per 100,000 for younger sailors. The rate in the Marine Corps was 19.3 per 100,000 for those aged 35–44, though it ranged from 11.9 to 14.5 for those who were younger (Hilton et al., 2009). Among soldiers, this trend is reversed: In 2006 and 2007, suicides were disproportionately concentrated among younger soldiers. In these years, almost half (49 percent in CY 2006 and 45 percent in CY 2007) of the Army suicides were under age 25, though only 40 percent of the total force falls in this age group (SRMSO, 2007, 2008). Between 2005 and 2007, suicide victims in the Air Force were disproportionately under 35 years of age, although, in 2008, suicide victims were disproportionately over age 35 (i.e., 38 percent of victims, compared with 27 percent of the entire Air Force) (Lichte, 2007; Loftus, 2008b; Kindt, 2009).

Racial and Ethnic Differences. There is a greater representation of nonwhite minorities in the military (30–36 percent of all military personnel, depending on component) than in the general population (in which three-quarters of the population report being white only) (U.S. Census Bureau, 2010; DoD, undated). Suicide rates in the United States have historically been higher among non-Hispanic whites and American Indian/Native Alaskans than among non-Hispanic blacks, Asian/Pacific Islanders, and Hispanics (CDC, 2010). While this general trend exists for both males and females, the differences are most pronounced among adults and the elderly, whereas racial and ethnic differences in sex-specific suicide rates are not as pronounced among those 10 to 25 years old (CDC, 2010). This corresponds to an increasing suicide rate among young African American males (Joe and Kaplan, 2001), and a higher prevalence of self-reported suicide attempts among Hispanic American high-school students than the national average of all high-school students (Eaton et al., 2006).

Some evidence suggests that suicides in the services reflect this general pattern of racial and ethnic differences. For example, between 1999 and 2007, suicide rates were highest in the Navy among Native Americans (19.3 per 100,000) and among non-Hispanic whites (11.9 per 100,000), whereas the rate in all other racial and ethnic groups was at or under 10 per 100,000. The rate in the Marine Corps for the same interval was highest among those with a race of "other or unknown" (25.0 per 100,000) and was also noticeably high among non-Hispanic whites (16.2 per 100,000) and Asians/Pacific Islanders (15.2 per 100,000) (Hilton et al., 2009). In 2006 and 2007, there was a slightly higher proportion of white suicide cases than in the Army overall (in 2006, 64 percent compared with 62 percent; in 2007, 67 percent compared with 63 percent) and fewer African American cases than in the Army overall (in 2006, 15 percent compared with 21 percent; in 2007, 11 percent compared with 20 percent). However, in both years in the Army, the proportion of suicide cases with an unknown or other racial or ethnic category was much higher than in the Army at large (in 2006, 7 percent compared with 3 percent; in 2007, 13 percent compared with 3 percent) (SRMSO, 2007, 2008). No rate is calculated among Native Americans who are currently placed in this "other" category yet who may have higher suicide rates that reflect trends in the general population.

Implications for DoD

Relative to the general population, the military is disproportionately male. Suicide rates are higher for males than females; thus, the expected suicide rate based on this demographic characteristic alone is higher among servicemembers than for the country as a whole, as is evident in the expected rate we calculated for Table 2.3.

Geographic Differences

We found no published estimates of military suicides in different geographic areas other than in theater (discussed later), which is particularly relevant for reservists, who tend to be geographically dispersed. Geographic differences in suicide rates exist in the civilian population. Suicide is more prevalent in the western United States: Alaska and Nevada have the highest suicide rates, while New Jersey has the lowest rate, though, in aggregate, the central states tend to have the lowest rates of suicide (Goldsmith et al., 2002). County-specific estimates indicate that the rate of suicide is higher in less densely populated (i.e., rural) counties, a trend that holds even after adjusting for county-level differences in age, sex, and race distributions (Goldsmith et al., 2002). However, there are areas in the West that are lower than the national average and areas in the central United States that are higher than the national average, though what distinguishes these areas remains unknown (Goldsmith et al., 2002).

Implications for DoD

We found no published information on recent suicides among military personnel as a function of geography. However, geographic variability may affect suicide rates in the military, since servicemembers are not uniformly dispersed throughout the United States.

Temporal Differences

Between 1991 and 2001, the suicide rate in the general population decreased for both sexes, at which point it remained constant for males, although, between 2001 and 2006, it increased among females (CDC, 2010). Historical evidence also suggests that suicide rates correlate with macroeconomic conditions: During economic downturns, there is evidence that the suicide rate increases (Wasserman, 1984). This may be due to a strong association between individual unemployment and suicide (Platt, 1984); however, there is not a strong correlation between the national unemployment rate and the U.S. suicide rate (Leenaars, Yang, and Lester, 1993).

In Figures 2.3–2.7, we present the suicide rates by year for each service along with the 95-percent confidence intervals we calculated as described earlier in the section "Variability in Rate Estimates." As shown in Figure 2.3, for DoD as a whole, there is some evidence that the suicide rate in CY 2008 was higher than the annual rate between CYs 2001 and 2005, as well as in CY 2007 relative to the average rate for CYs 2001 through 2008. The suicide rate in DoD for CY 2007 was higher than in CYs 2001 and 2002. In the Army, the suicide rates for CYs 2006 and 2007 were higher than in 2001 and 2004, and the rate in CY 2008 was higher than it was between CYs 2001 and 2005, as well as higher than the average rate for CYs 2001

Figure 2.3
Department of Defense Suicide Rates, Calendar Years 2001–2008

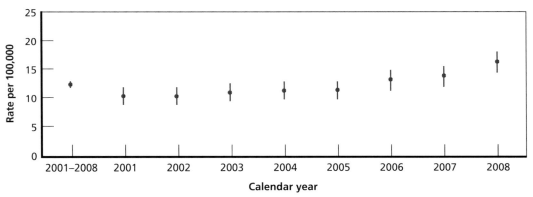

Figure 2.4
Army Suicide Rates, Calendar Years 2001–2008

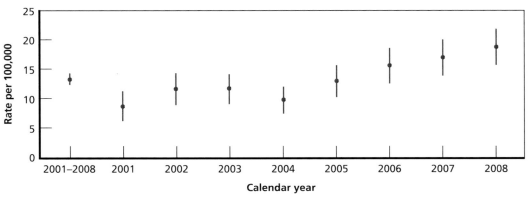

Figure 2.5
Navy Suicide Rates, Calendar Years 2001–2008

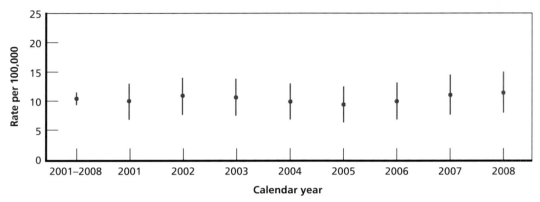

Figure 2.6
Air Force Suicide Rates, Calendar Years 2001–2008

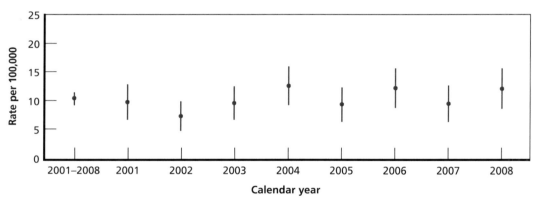

through 2008. In none of the other services was there evidence of differences across years. Thus, the data show only a few changes over time in terms of statistically significant differences.

Figure 2.7
Marine Corps Suicide Rates, Calendar Years 2001–2008

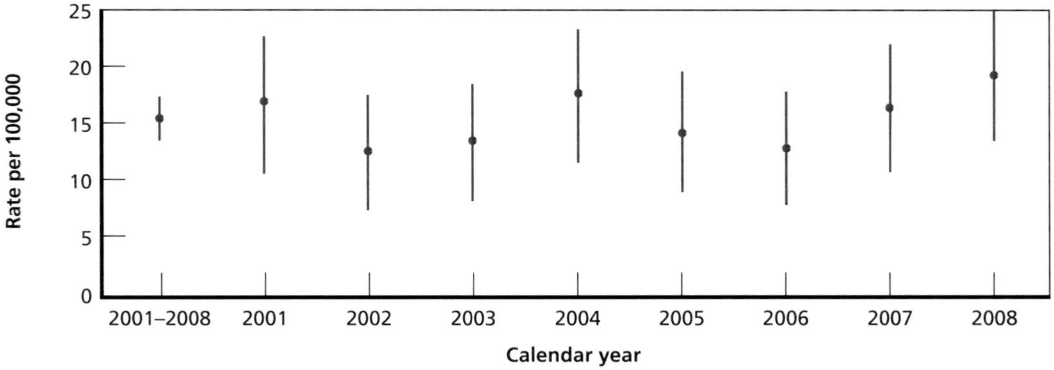

RAND *MG953-2.7*

Implications for DoD

Accounting for sampling error, there is evidence that the suicide rate in 2008 was higher than it was between 2001 and 2005 across DoD, and particularly in the Army.

There is reason to suspect that the national suicide rate may also be shifting, particularly since suicide is inversely correlated with economic conditions and the United States is currently experiencing a significant economic downturn. Data are not yet available to confirm this.

Military-Specific Characteristics

Rank Differences. Rank is confounded with age, so one would expect that differences in rank reflect the differences in age. This appears to be the case in the Army: In 2006 and 2007, 89 percent and 90 percent, respectively, of suicides were among enlisted personnel, who accounted for only 84 percent of the total force in both years. Among enlisted soldiers, suicides were disproportionately concentrated among echelons 1–4 (E1–E4s) relative to E5–E9s (SRMSO, 2007, 2008). This same pattern is also seen among the Navy and Marine Corps: Between 1999 and 2007, the suicide rate per 100,000 in the Navy was 11.3 for enlisted personnel and 7.1 for officers; in the Marine Corps, it was 15.4 for enlisted and 7.8 for officers (Hilton et al., 2009). Patterns by rank in the Air Force have been inconsistent: In 2005–2006, suicide victims in the Air Force were disproportionately ranked E1–E4 (47 percent of victims relative to 33 percent of airmen); in 2007, suicide victims were disproportionately E5–E6 (50 percent of victims relative to 35 percent of airmen) and, in 2008, were disproportionately E4s (22 percent compared with 15 percent) (Lichte, 2007; Loftus, 2008b; Kindt, 2009).

Component Differences. As mentioned previously, current DoD suicide estimates exclude nonactivated reservists. However, some reservists are included in the DoD estimates: all active National Guard reserve (full-time support personnel), activated Guard and reservists, and all Guard and reserve members who die by suicide en route to or during (1) initial active-duty training (boot camp and entry-level training), (2) two-week annual training, or (3) weekend inactive-duty training. While there are estimates across services of the proportion of active-duty suicides from the RC, we found no estimate of the suicide rate among activated reservists versus members of the active component.

Deployment. Since 2003, data have been collected on suicides that occur during an individual's deployment (Figure 2.8). The majority of U.S. forces deployed to Iraq and Afghanistan are soldiers and marines, so more suicides are expected to occur in theater among these personnel than among others. This is essentially the case. While few sailors and airmen killed themselves during deployment, approximately 30 percent of Army suicides since 2003 occurred in theater, and between 15 and 20 percent of suicides among marines since 2004 occurred in theater. The Army has also published data in its 2006 and 2007 ASER summary reports that indicate that at least 38 percent of suicides in CY 2006 and 39 percent of suicides in CY 2007 had no reported history of deployment (SRMSO, 2007, 2008).

Figure 2.8
Proportion of Suicides Occurring in Theater, Operation Enduring Freedom and Operation Iraqi Freedom

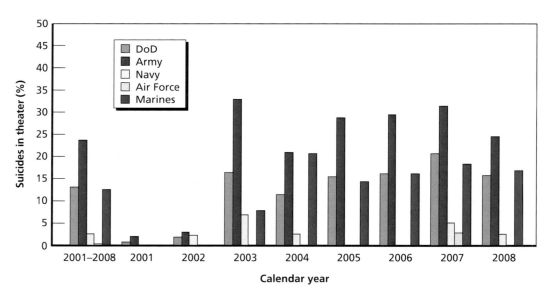

SOURCE: Mortality Surveillance Division, Armed Forces Medical Examiner (as of April 1, 2010).
RAND *MG953-2.8*

There is interest in the impact of multiple deployments on suicide, but, to date, there is insufficient evidence indicating the association. On the one hand, it has been suggested that multiple deployments may increase the risk of mental disorders, one of the strongest risk factors for suicide. On the other hand, a purported "healthy warrior effect" suggests that those able to deploy multiple times reflect a subset of warriors uniquely healthy and resilient to developing mental health problems or exhibiting suicidal behaviors (Haley, 1998).

Implications for DoD

While suicides disproportionately concentrate among lower ranks across the services, differences are not great, and suicides occur among all ranks.

A substantial proportion of suicides in the Army and Marine Corps occur in theater, stressing the need for suicide prevention for deployed personnel.

No research has yet been performed to estimate the proportion of suicides attributable to deployment, or the impact of multiple deployments on suicide.

Cause: Who Might Be at Risk of Dying by Suicide?

How Are Risk Factors Identified?

In trying to identify those factors that place an individual at risk for experiencing a health outcome, epidemiologists generally employ one of two study designs: cohort studies and case-control studies. Cohort studies are prospective in nature: Information on potential risk factors is collected at a single or multiple points of time for a sample of individuals, and these individuals are followed over time to see who does and who does not experience the outcome (e.g., death by suicide). The second strategy is a case-control study and is retrospective. Persons with the disease outcome of interest (cases) and a group without this outcome (controls) are surveyed, or researchers abstract previously collected data (e.g., from medical records) for both groups to determine whether the cases are more or less likely to have certain attributes than the controls. Case-series studies, such as the summary ASERs, are a third type of study that do not have a specified control group: This type of study is descriptive in nature and does not allow researchers to test directly whether certain factors are more common among suicide cases than among those who did not die by suicide.

Both cohort and case-control approaches are challenging when the disease outcome of interest is suicide. As mentioned previously, suicide is rare: The rate in the adult population hovers at around 10 per 100,000. The sample required to detect significant risk factors for suicide in a cohort study is large and, in most cases, cost-prohibitive. However, prospective studies following cohorts of groups at increased risk of suicide, such as psychiatric patients (see "Intrapersonal Correlates of Suicide: Mental and Substance-Use Disorders" in the next section), do provide some unique insights, though only among this population. The case-control approach thus may be a more attractive option, though it too carries with it unique challenges. Practically, it is impossible to survey suicide cases, since the subjects are all deceased. Thus, researchers using this approach have two options: use of data previously captured in administrative records alone or psychological autopsies. Psychological autopsies too use administrative records but involve interviewing key informants about the events leading up to the suicide, circumstances of the death (e.g., method), and other pertinent risk factors, such as psychopathology, family history of suicide and psychopathology, social functioning, personality characteristics, life stressors, history of treatment, physical health status, socioeconomic background and family background, and communication of suicidal intent. These interviews are optimally conducted between two to six months after an individual's death (Goldsmith et al., 2002). The control groups to which suicide cases are compared can be persons living in the community or those living in the community with evidence of mental disorder, but they can also be decedents who died from other causes. A proposed research collaboration between the U.S. Army and NIMH aims to adopt both prospective and case-control studies in the overarching research plan.

In the face of these challenges, researchers often expand their investigations to identify correlates and risk factors of suicide attempts or suicide ideation. Such inquiries provide insight into actual suicide because nonfatal attempts are the strongest predictors of completed suicide. However, the majority of those who die by suicide do so at their first attempt, and most of those who make a nonfatal attempt do not go on to die by suicide (see "Intrapersonal Correlates of Suicide: Prior Suicide Attempts"). Although it is obvious that fatal and nonfatal suicide attempts differ by definition with respect to lethality, some propose that those who make nonfatal attempts also differ from those who complete their suicide attempts, with respect to intent. Thus, suicide ideation and attempts are related to suicide deaths, though they should not be mistaken as proxies for suicide deaths.

Notwithstanding these research challenges, certain correlates of suicide have been identified. When there is evidence that the factor preceded the suicide outcome, it meets criteria to be deemed a risk factor (Kraemer et al., 1997). We describe correlates and risk factors of suicidal behavior in the following domains: intrapersonal, external, and social.

> ## Implications for DoD
>
> Epidemiologic studies produced by each service have thus far primarily been case-series reports that describe characteristics of those who have died by suicide and do not employ a control group.
>
> A 2008 collaboration between NIMH and the U.S. Army will prospectively follow a cohort of Army soldiers with a specific goal of learning more about suicidal behaviors. This type of study has the potential to contribute significantly to understanding suicide in the Army and to the field of suicide epidemiology more broadly.

Intrapersonal Correlates of Suicide

Prior Suicide Attempts. The majority of those who die by suicide die on their first attempt. In a retrospective study of suicides that occurred over 12 months in Finland, psychological autopsies revealed that 56 percent occurred as an individuals' first suicide attempt (Isometsa and Lonnqvist, 1998). However, this still implies that, in that year, 44 percent of deaths by suicide occur on an individual's subsequent suicide attempt. Prospective studies based on persons hospitalized for nonfatal suicide attempts provide evidence that risk of dying by suicide is greater among these individuals than it is in the general population. Within ten years of being hospitalized for a suicide attempt, close to 5 percent of New Zealanders died from another attempt (Gibb, Beautrais, and Fergusson, 2005); within 40 years of being hospitalized for self-poisoning, 15 percent of a sample of Finns eventually died by suicide (Suominen et al., 2004). Across studies, individuals with a history of suicide attempts have a 40- to 50-fold elevated risk of dying by suicide (Harris and Barraclough, 1997). Thus, although the majority of suicide deaths occur on individuals' first attempts and the majority of those who make nonfatal attempts do not go on to die by suicide, a prior suicide attempt is the strongest predictor of subsequent death by suicide.

Mental and Substance-Use Disorders. Psychological autopsies can yield valid psychiatric diagnoses among decedents (Kelly and Mann, 1996). Such studies indicate that approximately 90 percent of those who die by suicide have evidence of a mental disorder; case-control studies indicate that this compares with a rate of 27 percent among (mostly living) controls (Cavanagh, Carson, et al., 2003). Case-control studies conducted on adolescents and young adults indicate that 47 to 74 percent of suicides could be attributed to mental disorders, primarily affective or mood disorders (i.e., disorders that affect mood and influence thoughts, behaviors, and emotions), signaling to these authors that at least half the suicides among this population could be avoided with "completely effective treatment, or prevention, of mental disorders" (Cavanagh, Carson, et al., 2003). This has also led one leading researcher to propose that "suicide is generally a complication of a psychiatric disorder" (Mann, 2002), though two of the experts we interviewed disagree with this assessment and consider suicide a phenomenon separate from mental illness (see Chapter Three).

Certain mental disorders that carry an increased risk of suicide, such as schizophrenia (Tsuang, Woolson, and Fleming, 1980) and borderline personality disorder (Linehan, Rizvi, et al., 2000), are of minimal concern among military personnel. This is because many learning, psychiatric, and behavioral disorders are cause for rejection for appointment, enlistment, or induction into military service (National Research Council, 2006). Such rejection can be early on in the recruiting process, as well as during the early periods of initial training when enlisting in the service. However, the continuing deployment of U.S. military personnel to war zones in Iraq and Afghanistan has highlighted the emergence of specific mental health concerns that are relevant to this population: depression, anxiety disorders (including posttraumatic stress disorder, or PTSD), and harmful substance use and associated disorders. It is also relevant that we consider along with these mental health concerns psychiatric comorbidity (i.e., having more than one psychiatric disorder) and head trauma (e.g., traumatic brain injury, or TBI). We discuss the relationship of each with suicide.

Depression. Depression is a mood disorder characterized by feeling sad and blue for a period lasting more than two weeks, and with the result that such feelings interfere with a person's daily life. Among active-duty military personnel, just over 20 percent in 2005 and 2008 reported symptoms that, while not necessarily meeting diagnostic criteria for depression, indicate probable need for further clinical evaluation (Bray, Hourani, et al., 2006; Bray, Pemberton, et al., 2009). Among a sample designed to be representative of military personnel previously deployed to Iraq in support of OIF or Afghanistan in support of OEF, including reservists and those separated, 13.7 percent met criteria for probable major depression (Schell and Marshall, 2008).

Psychological autopsy studies indicate that depression is the most common mental disorder seen in suicide decedents with a history of mental illness (Cavanagh, Carson, et al., 2003). In cohort studies, persons with major depression have around 20 times the risk of dying by suicide (Harris and Barraclough, 1997). However, it is believed that only 4 percent of persons with depressive disorders will die by suicide—much higher than a rate of 0.01 percent in the general population but still a risk factor with limited predictive power (Goldsmith et al., 2002).

Anxiety, Including PTSD. There are eight distinct anxiety disorders classified in the *Diagnostic and Statistical Manual of Mental Disorders*, each of which is characterized by extreme symptoms of anxiety or fear. Thirteen percent of active-duty military personnel meet probable diagnostic criteria for generalized anxiety disorder (Bray, Hourani, et al., 2006). Of more recent concern since U.S. involvement in OIF and OEF, however, is the proportion of military personnel who screen positive for PTSD. PTSD is an anxiety disorder that may result after a person experiences a traumatic event. Exposure to such events is heightened during deployment to war zones. A recent survey designed to be representative of previously deployed U.S. military personnel, including reservists and those separated, indicates that 14 percent met probable diagnostic criteria for PTSD (Schell and Marshall, 2008). The prevalence of PTSD among U.S. military personnel has relevance to the proportion at increased risk for suicide, because community-based surveys indicate that persons with PTSD are more likely than those with any other anxiety disorder to report past suicide attempts and ideation (Kessler, Borges, and Walters, 1999; Sareen et al., 2005). A psychological autopsy study also revealed that Vietnam veterans who died by suicide were more likely to have PTSD than those who died in motor-vehicle crashes (Farberow, Kang, and Bullman, 1990). However, the proportion of those with PTSD, or any other anxiety disorder, who go on to die by suicide is unknown.

Substance Use and Associated Disorders. There is an elevated risk of death by suicide among persons with substance-use disorders as well as among heavy users of alcohol and other drugs. Psychological autopsy studies indicate that the median rate of substance abuse comorbid with a mental disorder among suicide decedents is approximately 38 percent, whereas the rate among (mostly living) controls is approximately 13 percent (Cavanagh, Carson, et al., 2003). Case-control studies also indicate that 23–46 percent of suicides among young adults and adolescents can be attributed to mental health disorders comorbid with substance abuse (Cavanagh, Carson, et al., 2003). Across cohort studies, there are more deaths by suicide than would be expected among persons with alcohol- or opioid-use disorders, intravenous drug users, those who use multiple psychoactive substances, and those who drink heavily. The magnitude of increased risk ranges from threefold (among heavy drinkers) to 17-fold (among those who use multiple drugs) (Wilcox, Conner, and Caine, 2004).

Case series of suicides indicate that between 28 and 53 percent of suicides are alcohol related, depending on the population being studied, and that between 20 and 30 percent of those who die by suicide are legally intoxicated at the time that they died (Goldsmith et al., 2002). Males under 50 who die by suicide are the suicide completers who are most likely to be intoxicated at the time of death (Hayward, Zubrick, and Silburn, 1992).

Heavy alcohol use remains a problem among military personnel. In the military, less than 5 percent of active-duty personnel report illicit drug use, likely due to DoD's urinalysis drug testing program. However, approximately 20 percent of servicemembers report heavy alcohol use (defined as drinking five or more drinks per typical drinking occasion at least once per week over the 30 days before being administered the survey), a proportion that has, for the most part, remained unchanged over the past 25 years (Bray and Hourani, 2007). There is also some evidence that those who have deployed in support of OIF and OEF are at increased risk of problem alcohol use upon returning from their deployment (Hoge, Auchterlonie, and Milliken, 2006; Jacobson et al., 2008). Screenings among those previously deployed indicate that 12 percent of deployed soldiers from the active component and 15 percent of deployed soldiers from the RC or National Guard reported using more alcohol than they intended to use, wanting or needing to cut down on their drinking, or both (Milliken, Auchterlonie, and Hoge, 2007).

Psychiatric Comorbidity. A strong body of evidence suggests that having more than one psychiatric disorder increases the likelihood of dying by suicide. In one study using psychological autopsies of 229 suicides in one year in Finland, 93 percent of victims were classified as having an axis I disorder (i.e., clinical disorder) and 88 percent had an axis I disorder with comorbidity (Henriksson et al., 1993). A separate study found that 57 percent of those who made serious suicide attempts had two or more psychiatric disorders and that the likelihood of having attempted suicide increased with increasing psychiatric morbidity (Beautrais et al., 1996). While estimates of comorbidity of psychiatric disorders among military personnel are rare, a nationally representative survey of military personnel who had served in OIF or OEF estimated that 3.5 percent had comorbid depression with PTSD (Schell and Marshall, 2008).

Head Trauma/TBI. Evidence also indicates that persons with concussions, cranial fractures, and cerebral contusions or traumatic intracranial hemorrhages each had at least three times the incidence rate of suicide mortality of the general population after adjusting for age and sex (Teasdale and Engberg, 2001). Other studies have found associations between self-reported suicide ideation and attempts and TBI (Hibbard et al., 1998). Among clinical samples of patients with TBI, between 18 and 26 percent report having attempted suicide or thought about killing themselves (Simpson and Tate, 2002, 2005). TBI is of particular concern among deployed military personnel who may sustain blast or other concussive injuries as a result of an explosion or blast of an improvised explosive device (IED) (Warden, 2006). Defining TBI in epidemiologic surveys is an emerging field, and current estimates among deployed personnel suggest that TBI prevalence ranges from 8 percent to 20 percent (Hoge, McGurk, et al., 2008; Schell and Marshall, 2008; Vasterling et al., 2006). Lasting impairments as a result of TBI remain unknown.

Psychological Correlates. Although mental and substance-use disorders are common among those who die by suicide, the majority of persons with such disorders do not go on to die this way. Thus, researchers have conducted studies to see how persons with the same mental disorders differ with respect to a history of suicide attempts (Mann et al., 1999) and eventual death by suicide (G. Brown, Beck, et al., 2000). Of those constructs that have been studied, three categories tend to be most clearly referenced with respect to suicidal behaviors: hopelessness, aggression and impulsivity, and problem-solving deficits.

Hopelessness. Of all psychological correlates, both statelike (i.e., chronic) and traitlike (i.e., acute) hopelessness are the only ones with a substantial body of evidence linking them with suicide. Whether traitlike or statelike, hopelessness is most commonly assessed with the Beck Hopelessness Scale, which measures hopelessness across three domains: feelings about the future, loss of motivation, and expectations (Beck and Steer, 1988). In studies that control for symptoms of depression and other mental disorders, as well as those conducted among psychiatric outpatients and inpatients, those who self-report higher levels of hopelessness are more likely to die by suicide (McMillan et al., 2007).

Aggression and Impulsivity. Some evidence links impulsivity and aggression with suicide, though most of this research is based on retrospective studies. For example, among a sample of 347 patients in a psychiatric hospital, those who had higher levels of impulsivity or aggression were more likely to report having attempted suicide (Mann et al., 1999). Some studies have failed to find this association, however, which suggests to one group of researchers that impulsivity is a factor in only a subset of all suicides (Wenzel, Brown, and Beck, 2009), including possibly those that also involve acute alcohol intoxication. Military personnel are generally more impulsive and appear more predisposed to take risks: Forty-six percent of active-duty military personnel are classified as having high levels of impulsivity, compared to less than 15 percent of civilian adults assessed ten years earlier (Bray, Pemberton, et al., 2009; Cherpitel, 1999).

Problem-Solving Deficits. Researchers propose that problem-solving deficits can both create stress and impede a person's ability to cope with stressful situations, which, in turn, may lead to suicide (Wenzel, Brown, and Beck, 2009). No prospective studies have yet linked problem-solving deficits with suicide, though such an association is seen consistently in cross-sectional studies that link problem-solving deficits with self-reports of suicide ideation (Rudd, Rajab, and Dahm, 1994) and a history of suicide attempts (Pollock and Williams, 2004).

Genetics. It is now widely accepted that suicide has a genetic component. Evidence of a genetic component comes from three different types of studies. First, those with a family member who has died by suicide are at increased risk of dying from suicide themselves (Brent and Mann, 2005). Second, there is higher concordance of suicide among monozygotic twins, who share close to 100 percent of the same genetic makeup, than among dizygotic twins, who share only 50 percent (Fu et al., 2002; Glowinski et al., 2001; Roy, 2001; Statham et al., 1998). Last, the likelihood of suicide is greater among the biological parents of adoptees who have died by suicide than in biological relatives of control adoptees, even after controlling for psychiatric disorders (Schulsinger et al., 1979). As of yet, the specific genetic components of suicide are unknown, and investigating the contribution of genetics to suicide remains an important field of research.

Neurobiology. Mann (2002) reviews findings from brain imaging and other novel studies to highlight neurobiologic changes that may increase individual risk for dying by suicide. Two neurotransmitters deserve special attention. Serotonin modulates human mood, anger, and aggression, while norepinephrine (which also acts as a stress hormone) affects attention and response actions, including the "fight-or-flight" response in humans. Studies show alterations in both serotonergic and noradrenergic systems among suicide victims, and continued research in this area is considered important for helping clinicians prevent suicide among persons with mental disorders.

Implications for DoD

Mental disorders and harmful substance use are linked with suicide. There is evidence that those who deploy are at risk for developing certain of these conditions (i.e., PTSD) and behaviors (i.e., binge drinking). Thus, without intervention and management of these conditions among afflicted individuals, one would expect the number of suicides in the military to increase.

The collaborative study between NIMH and the Army could help identify the risk of suicide among military personnel across multiple risk factors, and may also provide important information on psychological, genetic, and neurobiologic correlates of suicide.

External Risk Factors

History of Physical or Sexual Abuse. One retrospective study using psychological autopsies found that self-reports of past abuse was associated with suicide (Brent, Baugher, et al., 1999), and a number of studies have linked past childhood abuse, particularly sexual abuse, with suicide attempts (Goldsmith et al., 2002; Paolucci, Genuis, and Violato, 2001; Santa Mina and Gallop, 1998). It is not yet well understood whether childhood trauma independently increases the risk of suicide (Molnar, Berkman, and Buka, 2001) or whether the association is explained completely by mental disorders that are more likely to develop among individuals who have experienced childhood trauma (Fergusson, Woodward, and Horwood, 2000). Brent and Mann (2005) propose that abuse may play a role in familial aggregation of suicide in addition to any genetic role.

Life Events, Precipitating Events, and Triggers. Stressors are thought to interact with vulnerabilities to lead to suicidal behaviors. Many studies have indicated that life events, particularly negative ones, are more prevalent among persons who die by suicide (Cavanagh, Owens, and Johnstone, 1999) or who have attempted suicide (Paykel, Prusoff, and Myers, 1975; Yen et al., 2005). For example, there is evidence of excess risk of suicide, particularly among males, following the death of a spouse or parent (Bunch, 1972; Bunch et al., 1971; Luoma and Pearson, 2002; MacMahon and Pugh, 1965). However, while evidence indicates that both specific events (Yen et al., 2005) and the number of adverse life events (Paykel, Prusoff, and Myers, 1975) are associated with suicide, recent literature suggests that it is more an individual's reaction to an adverse life event, which is a product of his or her vulnerability to suicide, that influences the risk of suicide following these events. Prior mental health problems (Yen et al., 2005) or history of suicide attempts (Joiner and Rudd, 2000) may influence how people respond to adverse events in their lives.

For military personnel, deployment can increase the risk of experiencing stressors either independently or by affecting servicemembers' mental health, which, in turn, leads to increased stress (that is, deployment can itself be stressful and it can lead to mental health conditions that could cause other kinds of stress). Karney and colleagues (Karney et al., 2008) provide a review of the literature highlighting the many stresses to which deployed personnel may be exposed upon returning from deployment, including deterioration in physical health; problems in relationships with children, spouses, and other family members; employment difficulties; and financial hardship.

Implications for DoD

DoD publications have focused on highlighting specific life events among servicemembers who die by suicide. There is evidence to suggest that particular life events may differentially increase the risk of suicide. However, until studies include a control group, it will be impossible to discern which events, if any, specifically increase the risk of suicide among servicemembers.

Societal Risk Factors

Firearm Access. Consistent evidence indicates that availability of firearms is positively correlated with suicide. Evidence comes primarily from ecological studies that have uncovered statistically significant associations between death by suicide and household firearm ownership (Matthew Miller, Lippmann, et al., 2007) and changes in suicides correlated with changes in household firearm ownership (Matthew Miller, Azrael, et al., 2006). Case-control studies have found that persons who died by suicide were more likely to live in homes with firearms than in matched living (Kellermann et al., 1992) and dead (Kung, Pearson, and Wei, 2005) controls. Military personnel have access to firearms, particularly when deployed, and are more likely to own a personal gun than are other members of the general population (Hepburn et al., 2007).

Implications for DoD

Given the availability of firearms to servicemembers, when a servicemember makes a suicide attempt, he or she may be more likely than others to choose to use a firearm, which is the most lethal means by which one can kill oneself.

Suicides of Others and Reporting of Suicides. There is evidence to indicate that a suicide has the potential to produce imitative suicides. Evidence of contagion, whereby one suicide leads to a subsequent suicide, comes from studies that have documented a clustering of suicides in close temporal or geographic proximity, exposure to media coverage of suicides, and exposure to suicidal peers (Insel and Gould, 2008). Theories to explain suicide contagion generally note that individuals, particularly youth, learn behavior by observing and modeling others' behavior and that characteristics of suicide victims (e.g., high status) as well as gains from suicide (e.g., notoriety) are most likely to be modeled (Insel and Gould, 2008). Neurobiologic evidence suggests that adolescents and young adults may be particularly vulnerable to imitation than older adults (Insel and Gould, 2008). Since one-third to one-half of military personnel are under 25 (DoD, undated), imitation may be of particular concern for servicemembers.

A sizable body of literature points to clustering of suicides among teenagers (Gould, 1990; Gould, Wallenstein, and Kleinman, 1990; Gould, Wallenstein, Kleinman, et al., 1990). However, less than 5 percent of all youth suicides are seen in clusters (Insel and Gould, 2008). Evidence of suicides clusters among adults is not strong, though one published study suggests some clustering of suicides among U.S. Navy personnel between 1983 and 1995 (Hourani, Warrack, and Coben, 1999). In addition, although not statistically tested, there is indication of recent possible suicide clusters in the military: four suicides among Army recruiters in an East Texas battalion in 2008 ("Army Will Investigate Recruiters' Suicides," 2008) and four suicides in a National Guard unit in North Carolina (Goode, 2009).

There is also evidence that media coverage of suicide, particularly coverage that lasts for a long time, is featured prominently, and is covered extensively in newspapers, is associated with increases in suicide (Gould, 2001). Evidence for other forms of media, such as television (Kessler, Downey, Milavsky, and Stipp, 1988; Kessler, Downey, Stipp, and Milavsky, 1989; Stack, 1990), and fictional accounts of suicide (Berman, 1988; Gould, Shaffer, and Kleinman, 1988; Phillips and Paight, 1987) are inconclusive (Pirkis, 2009). Further, the Institute of Medicine (IOM) suggests that media coverage interacts with underlying personal vulnerabilities for suicidal behavior and may not be an independent risk factor. It states that "form (headline, placement) and content (celebrity, mental illness, murder-suicide) . . . impact the likelihood of imitation" and highlight that "attractive models are more likely to cause imitation" (Goldsmith et al., 2002, p. 278), a point reiterated in a recent review on media effects on suicide (Pirkis, 2009). There are insufficient studies of suicides related to the Internet to draw sound conclusions, though case studies suggest an important role of this media as influencing suicidal behaviors: Some youth have used the Internet to learn ways to kill themselves, and there are some anecdotal reports of Internet-based clustering (Insel and Gould, 2008).

There are correlations between one's own suicidality and one's exposure to peers who have either died by or attempted suicide (see Insel and Gould, 2008). Although primarily seen among youth, there is also at least one study to indicate that, in Stockholm, males exposed to a coworker's suicide faced a three-fold risk of suicide themselves (Hedstrom, Liu, and Nordvik, 2008). Such correlations could indicate that one person influences another person's suicidality, or that persons more likely to engage in suicidal behaviors are also more likely to form relationships with each other (i.e., "assortative relating"). Support for modeling is seen, for example, in a longitudinal study of youth that suggests that, among people who had never attempted, those who reported having a friend attempt suicide were more likely themselves to report an attempt at a subsequent interview (Cutler, Glaeser, and Norberg, 2001). On the other hand, there is also some support for assortative relating: In one study, college students who choose to live together reported more-closely aligned suicidal thoughts and behaviors than those randomly assigned to live together (Joiner, Steer, et al., 2003).

The phenomenon of suicide contagion may lead some individuals to speculate that asking, in surveys or clinical settings, about suicide ideation or attempts could prompt individuals to make a suicide attempt. Parents may have this concern when such questions are asked in surveys administered to their children (Fisher, 2003; Santelli et al., 2003), and primary-care physicians may not ask about suicide ideation out of fear that it will lead to suicidal behavior (Michel, 2000). To date, however, there is no evidence to suggest that asking about suicide ideation or attempts leads to suicidal behavior (Gould, Marrocco, et al., 2005; Hall, 2002).

Implications for DoD

There is some indication of possible suicide clusters among military personnel.

There is no evidence that asking about suicide ideation or attempts increases the risk of suicide.

Mechanisms: Why Do People Kill Themselves?

Thus far, we have described factors that are correlated with suicidal behavior, as well as some that appear to increase individuals' risk of dying by suicide. Now, we turn to the rubric of *mechanism*, which refers to the process by which these factors might actually lead to suicide.

The stress-diathesis model provides a framework to interpret most of the current prominent theories that explain suicidal behavior. The model proposes that every individual has a level of diathesis, or vulnerability, for a disease outcome—in our case, suicide. The diathesis alone does not produce the outcome, but problems emerge when an individual encounters varying levels of stress. Those with high vulnerability for suicide may act with seemingly lower levels of stress, while those less vulnerable are likely to act only under higher stress levels (Zubin and Spring, 1977).

Current theories that explain suicide generally complement—rather than compete with—each other. They differ in the way in which diathesis and stress interact to prompt an individual to take his or her life. Understanding the mechanisms that explain suicide is important for clinicians who seek to develop and implement treatment protocols for suicidal patients. The three theories we describe in this section are those that the key informants we interviewed indicated to be the prevailing theories explaining suicide.

Suicidal Schema

Cognitive theory describes schemata as the "lenses through which people view the world" (Wenzel, Brown, and Beck, 2009). They are informed by "features of stimuli, ideas, or experiences used to organize new information in a meaningful way thereby determining how phenomena are perceived and conceptualized" (Clark, Beck, and Alford, 1999, p. 79). Schemata may lie dormant and then activate in the face of adversity or stress.

A model developed by Wenzel and Beck (2008) proposes that individuals have "dispositional vulnerability factors" (i.e., long-standing characteristics, such as impulsivity, that increase the likelihood of a suicidal act) that can be considered the components of diathesis. These factors activate negative schemata in the face of life stress, create stress in and of themselves, or influence one's interpretation of events during a suicidal crisis. In times of stress, the activation of a negative schema causes maladaptive thoughts, interpretations, judgments, and images that lead to emotional, physiological, or behavioral responses that bolster the negative schema, creating a maladaptive feedback loop. For most individuals, this in and of itself does not lead to suicide but may lead to the development of psychiatric symptoms and/or diagnoses.

For a person to attempt suicide, Wenzel and Beck (2008) propose, the maladaptive feedback loop must escalate to the point at which it activates a specific suicidal schema. They have hypothesized two such schemata: a trait-hopelessness suicide schema and an unbearability suicide schema. The trait-hopelessness schema is characterized by the processing of cues as negative expectancies toward the future; it is termed *trait hopelessness* because it is stable over time. The unbearability suicide schema is one in which life stressors accumulate to the point at which an individual perceives them and the associated distress as unbearable. Either of these schemata increases the likelihood that an individual will experience *state* hopelessness, or hopelessness at a particular moment.

When a person detects suicide-relevant cues in a period of state hopelessness, he or she has a more difficult time disengaging from this information. As a result, individuals become overwhelmed, and their attention becomes fixated on suicide. Each individual has his or her own threshold of tolerance, and this threshold is crossed when an individual determines that he or she cannot tolerate the experience and decides to take his or her life.

Suicidal Mode

Cognitive theory holds that personality is comprised of four systems: cognitive (i.e., thoughts), affective (i.e., mood), behavioral, and motivational. A mode is a proposed suborganization of each of these four systems: a network of thought, mood, and behavior in which each system is simultaneously activated when a person is confronted with a specific event or when attempting to reach a goal. Rudd (2004) proposes that a suicidal mode is characterized by specific cognitions (i.e., pervasive hopelessness), affect (i.e., mixed negative emotions), behaviors (i.e., death-related behaviors, such as planning for suicide or attempting suicide), and an aroused physiological system. When confronted with an external trigger, all four systems may activate, which results in a suicidal crisis. Activation of the suicidal mode varies from person to person based on his or her vulnerability, which determines the threshold required for the mode to be activated or the variety of triggers that might activate the mode.

Acquired Ability to Enact Lethal Self-Injury

In 2005, Joiner proposed the interpersonal-psychological theory of suicidal behavior. This theory holds that two conditions must be met for a person to die by suicide. First, people who die by suicide must want to die. Those who want to die must experience two psychological states: They must perceive themselves to be a burden and lack a sense of belonging (e.g., to family, society). Additionally, Joiner claims that they must also have acquired the ability to enact lethal self-injury. In essence, the theory proposes that a human's natural instinct to self-preserve needs to be assuaged in order for a person to engage in self-injurious behavior that typically involves much intense fear or pain. Joiner proposes that individuals may acquire such ability through prior experiences with bodily harm, including nonfatal suicide attempts or other injurious behavior (Joiner, 2005).

A number of studies provide empirical support for Joiner's theory. For example, acquired ability to enact self-injury is supported by research indicating that those with prior suicide attempts experience more-serious future suicidality (Joiner, Steer, et al., 2003), while perceived burdensomeness is supported by research finding that higher levels of burdensomeness in suicide notes of those who died by suicide than in notes by those who attempted but did not die (Joiner, Pettit, et al., 2001). The importance of failed belongingness among those who die by suicide is supported by numerous studies, including a finding that Norwegian mothers with more children have lower suicide rates than those with fewer children (Høyer and Lund, 1993; Joiner and Van Orden, 2008).

Conclusion

This chapter summarizes what is known about suicide among military personnel according to the first four rubrics of epidemiology: quantity, location, cause, and mechanism. We also identified research from the general literature pertinent to those interested in acquiring a better understanding of suicide among military personnel and preventing suicide in this population. The next chapter is devoted entirely to the fifth rubric: prevention and control.

CHAPTER THREE

Best Practices for Preventing Suicide

This chapter reviews information on the current status of suicide-prevention efforts relevant to the military context. We begin with a framework that describes the continuum of intervention activities and the ways in which they may be combined. We use existing published literature and expert opinion to describe current best practices along this continuum. We also highlight evidence, when it exists, that suggests that certain programs or formats could be detrimental and actually increase risk of suicide. We extract information seen as most pertinent to the prevention of suicide in the military and place it in text boxes to highlight those points. Finally, we conclude with an assessment of the general status of evidence for various approaches, and recommendations for future prevention programming based on these findings.

The Public Health Framework for Prevention

A public health framework classifies programs and policies designed to prevent diseases by the populations that they serve. Those that target the entire population are referred to as *universal* or *primary prevention*; those targeting selected groups based on a common risk factor are referred to as *selective* or *secondary prevention*; and programs delivered to individuals with detectable symptoms are referred to as *indicated prevention* (Mrazek and Haggerty, 1994). Although suicide is not a disease, we follow the convention of past research and describe suicide prevention using this organizational framework. However, a few exceptions are worth noting. First, we include dimensions of self-care (i.e., an individual's ability to limit adversarial situations, manage stress, and seek help) and environmental safety (i.e., limiting access to lethal means) that span across the entire continuum of prevention, from universal to indicated. Second, interventions designed for populations that share a certain risk factor (selected prevention) and those designed for individuals with detectable symptoms (indicated prevention) cannot be easily distinguished, so we discuss them together in this monograph. Third, we include a category of *postvention*, which refers to the way a death by suicide is handled by an organization or the media.

NIMH also acknowledged these unique features of suicide prevention and modified a framework of optimal mental health service mix originally developed by the World Health Organization (Schoenbaum, Heinssen, and Pearson, 2009). In this model, prevention programs are not clearly divided into universal, selected, and indicated, but instead are placed across a prevention continuum, with a dimension of self-care and environmental control that runs across the entire continuum as well. The framework describes primary prevention programs as delivered on a broad scale, for a relatively small cost per person, whereas treatment programs are delivered to few at high expense. This framework represents an ideal way to discuss the merits and limitations of the different prevention programs.

With respect to prevention, programs designated as involving best practices are those that contain an activity or set of activities that have been demonstrated through research or evaluation to achieve the stated goal. Adopting this definition, a best practice for suicide prevention would be supported by evidence demonstrating that a given program causally reduced suicides. Currently, only a handful of programs would meet this strict definition. The challenge in determining best practices for suicide prevention is due to the paucity of available data on the effectiveness of the programs. Programs to prevent deaths by suicide pose particular challenges to evaluation efforts:

- Base rates of the phenomenon under study (deaths by suicide) are low, which makes identification of meaningful effects difficult (see Chapter Two).
- Long time frames are necessary to observe prevention outcomes (i.e., reduction in suicides).
- It is difficult to classify and track suicides, and there is known variability in how suicides are classified (see Chapter Two).
- Better understanding of risk factors is needed. The lack of strong predictive power of known risk factors hampers efforts to focus on programs for high-risk groups.
- Many programs contain multiple components, making it difficult to discern the effective components or ingredients responsible for any observed effect.
- Measuring suicidal ideation, suicide attempts, or other suicidal behavior as a proxy for deaths by suicide is imperfect (see Chapter Two).

These challenges make the literature on effectiveness of suicide-prevention programs sparse, and conclusions that can be drawn from the literature tentative. Thus, our review of best practices in preventing suicide included a review of the published literature, as well as structured interviews with experts in the field, described in more detail in Chapter One. Our review of best practices does not attempt to be comprehensive but rather to highlight the most-promising practices observed in the empirical literature and expert opinion. For comprehensive reviews, see Goldsmith et al. (2002) and Mann (2005).

In this chapter, we discuss what the literature and experts consider to be the most-promising approaches for preventing suicide. While we categorize programs as universal or selected or indicated, it is important to note that many suicide-prevention programs may include elements from different parts of the continuum of prevention programs, and some are difficult to place on the continuum at all. Nonetheless, this framework still provides a useful way to discuss programs in terms of their targets and aims. Of particular importance is the fact that there is very little research on the "broad" end of the spectrum, in terms of what programs work for primary prevention. Rather, the bulk of the strong evidence about effectiveness concentrates at the selected or indicated prevention end of the spectrum, focusing on interventions or treatments for those deemed to be at increased risk for suicide or who have displayed past suicidal behavior.

Primary or Universal Prevention Programs

Primary prevention programs are those delivered at a population level (e.g., to every-one in a country, state, or school). Some efforts that fall into this domain are general health-promotion programs that may have suicide reduction as a benefit but are gener-ally not designed with suicide reduction as the primary goal. These efforts can include such things as substance-abuse prevention or general mental health promotion. For a concrete example, increases in the legal drinking age between 1970 and 1990 were related to reductions in suicides, as well as reductions in the number of deaths by motor-vehicle accidents (Birckmayer and Hemenway, 1999).

There are also specific suicide-prevention activities, generally falling into two categories: (1) those that raise awareness and teach skills and (2) those that provide screening and referral for mental health problems and suicidal behavior. Although the referral aspect could be considered a "selective" intervention, since it is only for those deemed to be at risk, we include screening efforts that target the whole population in this section, because they normally start with the entire population (e.g., school, mili-tary unit) rather than targeting specific individuals to begin with. We discuss each of these categories in turn.

Raising Awareness and Building Skills
For these programs, the general strategy is to enhance protective factors and reduce risk factors of suicide across a population. Most of the programs evaluated to date that fall into this category are school-based programs (e.g., high schools), and the ones that produce most sustained behavior change are those that are multidimensional, include health-promotion strategies and skill training, and are embedded in an envi-ronment containing trained, supportive adults (Goldsmith et al., 2002). Promising elements of these programs include training in the importance of youth telling adults

and seeking help for self or friends, and skill training (active-listening social skills, positive self-talk, situational-analysis empathy training, role playing, interrupting automatic thoughts, rehearsal and skill strengthening, and help-seeking). Programs differ in their approach in building these skills, from didactic presentations to role-plays to having youth train other youth. One such program is the Signs of Suicide® (SOS) program, which teaches students to "acknowledge, care, and tell" about suicide, and is similar to the Army's Ask, Care, Escort (ACE) and Navy's Ask, Care, Treatment (ACT) campaigns (described in Chapter Four and in Appendixes A and B). This program has demonstrated improvements in knowledge and attitudes about suicide, as well as reductions in self-reported suicide attempts by the students who received it (Aseltine et al., 2007), but results were based on anonymous surveys, so it is not clear whether the intervention had the desired impact on those who were most at risk (e.g., those absent from school). Another program that was implemented with first and second graders, the Good Behavior Game, demonstrated reduced suicide ideation and attempts at ages 19–21, even though the immediate targets of the program were to "socialize children for the student role" and to reduce aggressive and disruptive behavior (Wilcox, Kellam, et al., 2008).

Evaluations of other programs to date show some changes in knowledge and attitudes about suicide, but not reductions in actual deaths by suicide. Among these programs, the most promising appear to be those that include a focus on behavior change and that teach coping strategies, such as seeking social support, rather than on knowledge and attitudes alone (Guo and Harstall, 2004). This approach of building skills in a general population was endorsed by several of the experts interviewed.

Programs that only raise awareness do not seem to be helpful and may be detrimental, as can other short, didactic programs with no follow-up or continuity (Goldsmith et al., 2002), because they do not provide enough time to deal with the issues raised in the session. In particular, any universal prevention program that might inadvertently increase the stigma for those experiencing suicidal states was thought by experts to be potentially detrimental, since it could actually lead to more barriers to care for those in need. Beyond these general speculations (that programs including skill building would be most helpful and that those that increase stigma could be detrimental), there is very little information about what types of universal programs are to be recommended or the specific elements within each that are the active ingredients or most important to include. Thus, there is little information to guide new prevention efforts.

The Blue Ribbon Work Group on Suicide Prevention in the Veteran Population identified a few different universal or primary prevention programs already in use for veterans within the Veterans Health Administration (VHA). These include outreach to veterans at deployment and reintegration times, as well as embedding a suicide-prevention coordinator (SPC) in primary care to help increase awareness about suicide. The panel considered this a promising approach to suicide prevention and recommended ongoing evaluation of the program (Blue Ribbon Work Group on Suicide Prevention in the Veteran Population, 2008).

Screening and Referral

Several models exist for improving access to quality mental health care by providing screening within primary-care settings or other social settings. In these settings, patients and clients can be screened either for depression or for suicidal ideation or intent. In reviewing evidence for such screenings, it was concluded that screening adults for depression in primary care improves patient outcomes (Pignone et al., 2002). However, there is only limited evidence to guide clinical assessment and management of suicidal risk (Gaynes et al., 2004). Thus, the U.S. Preventive Services Task Force currently recommends that primary-care clinicians screen for depression, but it does not provide a recommendation for or against screening for suicide risk in primary care (U.S. Preventive Services Task Force, undated).

One model that educates physicians about how to recognize depression and assess for suicide risk was identified as an effective method of preventing suicide (Mann, 2005). For example, a program in Gotland, Sweden, trained physicians to recognize symptoms of depression and was associated with an increase in the number of diagnoses and treated depressed patients, along with reductions in suicide (Rutz, von Knorring, and Wålinder, 1989). However, the authors caution that additional follow-on sessions may be necessary. The need for specific training for clinicians was emphasized by one of the experts we interviewed, who explained that clinicians often do not receive adequate training to assess suicide risk under normal circumstances, so there is a need for special training efforts. Training for other types of professionals to serve in this role has not yet been evaluated.

Going beyond physician education alone, other efforts have put routine screening into place in primary care or other non–mental health settings. When screening programs are in place, it is essential that the screening be followed by enhanced care for those with an identified problem. Examples include collaborative care models for treating depression in primary care (Bruce, Ten Have, et al., 2004; Engel et al., 2008; Unützer et al., 2002) or other health-care settings, such as home health care for the elderly (Bruce, Brown, et al., 2007). Collaborative care models generally bring mental health expertise into these settings by means of training and expert consultation, as well as explicit linkages that are aimed at reducing barriers to behavioral health care. Often, a care manager is assigned to help the patient decide on the best course of treatment and to help navigate the system so that he or she accesses the most-appropriate resources. These interventions have been shown to be effective in reducing depression and, in one instance, in reducing suicidal ideation (Unützer et al., 2002).

An important caveat is that any efforts to screen or detect depression or suicidal ideation must be followed with access to quality mental health services, and repeated screening is necessary, since suicidal ideation and intent are episodic states (Goldsmith et al., 2002). In addition, two of the experts we interviewed cautioned that treatment of mental health problems as the sole means of reducing suicide was not well supported by the evidence and that suicidal behavior must be addressed separately as a distinct type of problem. However, other experts we interviewed who considered suicide to be a complication of mental illness countered this perspective. Still, detection and follow-up could occur in primary-care settings.

Screening for mental health problems and suicide risk has also been conducted among youths in school in the TeenScreen® program, and, more recently, this program has been extended to primary-care settings as well. The screening measures were evaluated and shown to identify youth at risk for mental health problems, most of whom were not previously known to have problems (Shaffer et al., 2004; SAMHSA, 2010). However, whether this screening program can lead to reduced suicidal behavior has not been evaluated.

The VA Blue Ribbon Panel examined current VHA efforts to conduct routine screening in primary care and generally looked favorably upon those strategies, with two exceptions. They noted some concerns about the exact screening measures and cut-offs used to flag individuals at risk and noted some deficiencies in protocols for when and how to remove the flags for individuals, due to lack of empirical evidence for each (Blue Ribbon Work Group on Suicide Prevention in the Veteran Population, 2008).

Selected or Indicated Suicide-Prevention Programs

Selected prevention programs are those that are delivered to groups that may be at elevated risk for suicidal behavior by virtue of some risk factor, such as having a mental health problem or because of known suicidal behavior or ideation. Indicated programs are designed for specific individuals who are known to be symptomatic for a given disease. However, since no symptoms have yet been uniquely identified with significant predictive power that lead to suicide (see Chapter Two), we combine these categories. A challenge for the military is determining what risk factors may be most pertinent to servicemembers. Together, civilian prevention programs in this area fall into one of two categories: those that target groups at high risk by virtue of a known risk factor (e.g., high-school dropout, mental illness) and those that work directly with suicide attempters who come to the attention of health providers because of their suicidal behavior. We discuss each in turn.

Interventions with High-Risk Groups

Suicide-prevention programs in this category target individuals who may never have displayed suicidal behavior but are known to have elevated risk for death by suicide. For example, while not necessarily a problem among military personnel, among youth, being a school dropout is associated with suicide risk as well as a host of other problems

(E. Thompson and Eggert, 1999). Thus, one school-based program targeted potential high-school dropouts. Called Reconnecting Youth™, this program consisted of support and skill training, and demonstrated significant decreases in suicide risk behaviors, depression, hopelessness, anger, and stress, as well as gains in self-esteem, personal control, and reported social support (Eggert, Thompson, et al., 1995).

As described in Chapter Two, mental illness is one of the strongest identified risk factors for suicide, leading one group of researchers to conclude that a large proportion of suicides could be avoided with "completely effective treatment, or prevention, of mental disorders" (Cavanagh, Carson, et al., 2003). There are selective prevention programs focused on serving those with mental health problems. While there is evidence that many individuals, both in the general population (Luoma, Martin, and Pearson, 2002) and in the military (SRMSO, 2007, 2008), have seen a mental health professional a short time before killing themselves, a review of public data on deaths from suicide determined that a common factor was a failure or breakdown in the *continuity of care* for mental health problems (Schoenbaum, Heinssen, and Pearson, 2009). Having a "chain of care" and "warm transfers" would prevent individuals from "falling through the cracks of the care system" and is seen as particularly important for individuals suffering from a mental health problem or experiencing suicidal ideation or intent. In the military context, it would mean ensuring smooth transitions between providers during transition times (e.g., moves, deployments, redeployment) so that there is always care available. Of particular note may be the need to transition from medications prescribed in theater upon return home. The concept provides an excellent framework for understanding some of the successful efforts that can guide suicide-prevention work within the continuum of selective and indicated prevention programs.

Part of an appropriate chain of care would be assurance that effective treatments are delivered for individuals with specific mental health problems, with or without known suicidal ideation or intent. These methods include medications, such as lithium for bipolar disorder (which may have limited applicability among military personnel, since those with bipolar disorder may be deemed unfit for duty) and selective serotonin-reuptake inhibitors (SSRIs) or other antidepressants (Blue Ribbon Work Group on Suicide Prevention in the Veteran Population, 2008; Goldsmith et al., 2002; Leitner, Barr, and Hobby, 2008) and psychotherapies for depression (Goldsmith et al., 2002). However, one expert noted that these empirically validated treatments have not usually been tailored or tested exclusively with suicidal patients. Nonetheless, data do exist for some of them that indicate reduced suicidal behavior at a group level among patients treated with them. Recent concern that SSRIs can increase the risk of suicide in those under the age of 25 has created a good deal of confusion among practitioners, and some reluctance to use them to treat depression in this age group. However, much of the evidence to date on this point is inconclusive, and such medications are still seen as beneficial overall in reducing depression and related suicidality at a population level (Brent, 2009).

An example of improvements in behavioral health comes from the Division of Behavioral Health Services of the Henry Ford Health System in Detroit, which implemented Perfect Depression Care. This initiative took recommendations directly from the IOM's (2006) Crossing the Quality Chasm report, focusing on four main activity areas (partnership with patients, clinical care, access, and information flow), and demonstrated a decrease in suicide by 75 percent (Coffey, 2007).

Implications for DoD

It is as yet unclear which risk factors should be targeted in military suicide-prevention efforts. Many learning, psychiatric, and behavioral disorders are cause for rejection for appointment, enlistment, or induction into military service (National Research Council, 2006). However, the stresses of deployment and combat exposure are known to increase risk for depression and PTSD. Research is needed to determine which higher-risk groups in the military may benefit from suicide-prevention programs.

Ensuring good access to high-quality care for those with mental health problems is a key part of suicide prevention, with an emphasis on continuity of care.

Interventions at the Time of Suicidal Ideation or Intent

Additional programs have been developed to intervene with individuals who come to the attention of "gatekeepers" when they are experiencing suicidal ideation or intent. Gatekeepers include such people as clergy, first responders, and employees in schools and work settings, such as the military. In some programs, peers may also be trained as gatekeepers. These programs typically teach people to identify those at risk for suicide and to take these individuals (or encourage them to go) to specific people, such as school counselors or social workers, who then help link the individual with mental health services. The keys of any gatekeeper training are the presence of quality services into which to refer individuals and that the gatekeepers know and trust those resources (Goldsmith et al., 2002; Schoenbaum, Heinssen, and Pearson, 2009).

The Question, Persuade, Refer program, or QPR, was demonstrated to improve knowledge, appraisals of efficacy, and service access but not suicide identification behaviors with students (Wyman et al., 2008). Exploration showed that secondary-school staff who increased in suicide identification behaviors were those who started out the program already talking to their students about suicide. Other examples of these programs include LivingWorks Applied Suicide Intervention Skills Training (ASIST) (Eggert, Randell, et al., 2007) and Suicide, Options, Awareness, and Relief

(Project SOAR) (King and Smith, 2000). Both of these programs demonstrated that the gatekeepers (e.g., school counselors) could learn the materials and skills taught (e.g., can demonstrate knowledge of the steps to take and can demonstrate competencies in simulations). However, one expert warned that the emphasis on training for gatekeeper models has thus far been on training individuals on how to give help to others but that there is not enough emphasis on how to ask for help. Presumably, individuals would need to be prepared to both offer and ask for help if a gatekeeper model is to work. Special efforts might be needed to overcome barriers to asking for help, which include barriers common among the general population (Kessler, Berglund, et al., 2001), as well as those that are particularly important to military personnel (Schell and Marshall, 2008) (see Table 3.1), and to find ways to fit this concept into the military culture and language. Strong stigma around mental health problems or mental health treatment in general as a barrier to seeking help was reiterated by experts we interviewed.

Hotlines offering support and referral are also common practices. The National Suicide Prevention Lifeline (NSPL), now triaging veterans to link them with a VA-trained staff member, has been evaluated in terms of the quality of responses but not in terms of its actual suicide-prevention effectiveness (Goldsmith et al., 2002; Gould, Kalafat, et al., 2007; Kalafat et al., 2007).

Inpatient hospitalization is a common measure for ensuring safety for an individual with intent to die by suicide but has not actually been demonstrated to work as a prevention tactic. It appears that hospitalization alone does not prevent suicide but rather that it is the interventions that are conducted while in the hospital or upon discharge that are key (Goldsmith et al., 2002). However, hospital stays are often too short to allow for specific interventions to be delivered. Similarly, "no-suicide" contracts between patients and health providers, in which patients agree, often in writing, not to harm themselves, are widely used (Michael Miller, Jacobs, and Gutheil, 1998) but have not been demonstrated to be effective when used on their own (Goldsmith et al., 2002).

How suicidal patients are assessed within the mental health system is another area in which to examine best practices. A few experts interviewed expressed skepticism about this key aspect of the model, stating that there is too much confidence placed

Table 3.1
Barriers to Mental Health Care in the General Population and Among Formerly Deployed Military Personnel

In the General Population (Kessler, Berglund, et al., 2001)	Among Formerly Deployed Military Personnel (Schell and Marshall, 2008)
Lack of perceived need	Negative career repercussions
Unsure about where to go for help	Inability to receive a security clearance
Cost (too expensive)	Concerns about confidentiality
Perceived lack of effectiveness	Concerns about side effects of medications
Reliance on self (desire to solve problem on one's own or thoughts that the problem will get better)	Preferred reliance on family and friends
	Perceived lack of effectiveness

in behavioral health-care professionals' ability to assess and manage a suicidal patient, when in fact most professionals do not have the requisite training to do so. Some protocols exist to describe how to determine risk level for a given patient (Raue et al., 2006) but have not yet been formally tested. Although there are known correlates of suicide attempts (see Chapter Two), none of these risk factors is a perfect predictor, and, thus, much is left to the subjective judgment of the assessor. Some instruments have been developed to aid in risk assessment, such as the Suicide Attempt Self-Injury Interview (Linehan, Comtois, Brown, et al., 2006). Further developments into an online version and modifications for the military are under way.

When suicidal patients access a crisis-intervention service, hotline, or emergency room, there are also models for how to use those contacts as "teachable moments" in addition to making a referral. Assessing patients for suicide risk and restricting their access to lethal means, such as firearms, is seen as a key element to intervention in these instances (Simon, 2007). For example, a promising approach identified by NIMH staff is Screening, Brief Intervention, and Referral to Treatment (SBIRT) (see SAMHSA, undated), which is utilized in many hospital and employment settings for alcohol abuse and other risky behaviors (Schoenbaum, Heinssen, and Pearson, 2009). A short protocol that uses safety planning as a crisis-intervention tool has been developed by Barbara Stanley and Gregory Brown, including a revision for veterans called SAFE VET (Stanley and Brown, 2008), though neither the original nor the adaptation has yet been evaluated. Another brief protocol that has been developed is the Collaborative Assessment and Management of Suicidality (CAMS) treatment that includes means restriction, developing crisis response, and building interpersonal connections (Jobes et al., 2005). However, it too requires evaluation.

A few studies support the concept of continued contact or outreach following a crisis or hospitalization for suicidal behavior or severe depression. Some of these programs have been proven to be successful, such as use of "caring letters" following hospital discharge, giving patients an emergency card, or using a suicide counselor to coordinate care following hospital discharge (Aoun, 1999; Morgan, Jones, and Owen, 1993; Motto and Bostrom, 2001). However, on balance, the findings are equivocal, with other studies finding no impact on rates of suicide ideation or attempts (Allard, Marshall, and Plante, 1992; Cedereke, Monti, and Öjehagen, 2002; Rotheram-Borus et al., 2000), and still others finding reductions on some aspects of suicidal behavior measured but not others (Carter et al., 2005, 2007; Vaiva et al., 2006). Thus, there is still a need for further evaluation to identify specific aspects of these interventions that make them successful under some circumstances but not others. One expert we interviewed suggested that more could be done within military units to ensure continuity of support from peers and commanders and that alienation or criticism from members of the unit might be particularly difficult for suicidal individuals to handle.

In addition to the interventions for behavioral health problems reviewed earlier, which do not focus specifically on suicidal behavior but rather on the mental health problems, two specific interventions target suicidal thoughts and behaviors directly. These models could be considered treatment, but they also prevent deaths by suicide among high-risk individuals. Both have been tested to some degree and have shown effectiveness:

- Dialectical behavior therapy (DBT) is a treatment developed for suicidal and parasuicidal behavior (also called suicide gestures, in which the intent is not death, but the means can be similar). Its developer considers it to be not a suicide-prevention program as much as it is a "life worth living" program. The treatment encourages patients to develop explicit reasons for living and targets skill building and safety planning. It is an intensive, one-year model and has shown reductions in suicide attempts among individuals displaying recent suicidal or self-injurious behavior who have borderline personality disorder (Linehan, Comtois, Murray, et al., 2006). Use of this method with individuals who do not have a personality disorder is not well tested to date.
- Second, cognitive therapy (CT) can help when based on theories of a suicidal schema (see Chapter Two) that focuses on specific thoughts and behaviors that are part of the individual's acute hopelessness state and selective attention that are hypothesized to form the suicidal state. Along with other forms of treatment (e.g., intensive case management and other treatments as necessary), this six-month treatment has been shown to reduce suicide attempts among prior attempters (G. Brown, Ten Have, et al., 2005). However, these results have not yet been replicated.

These intensive interventions have not yet been tested in the military context, but some efforts are currently under way. David Rudd is testing a CT model in the Army, and Marjan Holloway is testing a modification of Brown's model among inpatient suicide attempters at Walter Reed Army Medical Center. Results of these studies will be informative on the usefulness of the interventions in the military context. While the interventions carry the best available evidence in suicide prevention in the civilian context, they are time-intensive (and therefore expensive) interventions that need to be delivered by trained providers.

Implications for DoD

Stigma and lack of confidentiality may inhibit disclosure of suicidal ideation or intent, limiting the success of gatekeeper models or uptake of mental health services.

Gatekeeper models and hotlines have emphasized how to *offer* help but could benefit from more emphasis on how to *ask* for help.

Gatekeeper models and hotlines require high-quality services to back them up, including having clinicians prepared to conduct state-of-the-art risk assessment, brief interventions, and treatment if required. Gatekeepers also must trust the resources that are available for referral.

It is unclear the extent to which mental health professionals are prepared to handle suicidal individuals appropriately, and similar concerns exist for other professionals who may be engaged in the chain of care (e.g., clergy).

Risk-assessment tools are being developed, but not yet evaluated, in the civilian sector. Similar tools would be valuable if tailored to military personnel and should be accompanied by quality-assurance processes.

The risk-assessment phase offers the opportunity to offer brief intervention, such as CAMS and the SAFE VET protocol, but these still need evaluation.

Proven intervention techniques (CT and DBT) for those with known suicidal behavior need to be evaluated in the military context and made available through regular systems of care (e.g., MTFs, TRICARE).

Continuity by means of letters and phone calls following suicidal behavior has mixed support, but these modes of communication are inexpensive and may be worth testing in the military context. Focus on positive interpersonal connections and continuity within units may be useful.

Environmental Safety or Means Reduction

Evidence supports the use of means reduction or enhancements to safety on all parts of the continuum in suicide prevention, from universal efforts to those targeted at suicide attempters or those with imminent intent. This practice identifies the means by which people in a particular population kill themselves and then how to make these means less available. Examples of such initiatives include policies that restrict access to firearms to prevent self-inflicted gunshot wounds, use of blister packs for lethal medications to prevent intentional overdoses, bridge safeguards to prevent fatal falls, and constructing shower-curtain rods so as to prevent fatal hangings. One retrospective study of suicide cases among Irish military troops revealed that availability of lethal means was a prominent factor among cases (Mahon et al., 2005). Firearms are the most common method of suicide in the military: Between 1999 and 2007, firearms were used in 51 percent of Navy suicides and 63 percent of suicides among marines (Hilton et al., 2009). Firearms were also used in 71 percent of Army suicides in 2006 and 63 percent in 2007 (SRMSO, 2007, 2008). The VA Blue Ribbon panel highlighted recent efforts for veterans that include child-oriented attention to home gun safety (e.g., safe storage of ammunition and gun-safety locks), as well as modifications to door hinges to reduce deaths by hanging among patients (Blue Ribbon Work Group on Suicide Prevention in the Veteran Population, 2008).

Implications for DoD

Reducing access to lethal means of suicide is a proven practice for reducing suicides and is underutilized in the military.

Attention to private gun ownership and home gun safety may be important.

Peers, gatekeepers, and health-care professionals engaged in suicide-prevention efforts should remove or restrict access to firearms, as well as promote safe and separate storage of ammunition and use of safety locks.

Identification of other prominent means of death can lead to further means-reduction efforts.

Postvention

The concept of postvention, or efforts to handle deaths by suicide as they occur so as to prevent future suicides, has also received some attention in the civilian best-practice literature. These efforts primarily have to do with training for the media to reduce the possibility of imitative suicides (discussed in Chapter Two) and include guidelines on reporting of suicides, such as not glorifying the death or describing the means by which suicide victims ended their lives (Pirkis et al., 2006). For instance, the CDC offers guidelines (O'Carroll, Mercy, and Steward, 1988), and these have been utilized for contagion containment to reduce suicide deaths within a community (Hacker et al., 2008). In addition, promising postvention programs are being developed and implemented that involve bringing both civilian and military stakeholders together to develop a comprehensive plan that includes clearly defined roles and responsibilities for each organization in the event of a suicide (Norton, 2009). While most of the experts we interviewed felt that postvention was a critical component of preventing suicide, there is limited empirical evidence linking these efforts with actual reductions in suicides (Goldsmith et al., 2002).

Implications for DoD

Developing a response to suicides and suicide attempts is a critical component of suicide prevention, and best practices exist. These include clearly defined roles and guidelines for reporting suicides.

Media coverage of military deaths by suicide should follow best practices for media.

Integrated Programs

Many initiatives to prevent suicide are integrated approaches that simultaneously implement coordinated universal and selected or indicated prevention components. Many of these programs also include a strong component of restricting access to lethal means, particularly restricting access to firearms. Such programs are seen primarily at the state or national level, although a current effort under way includes four European Union countries (Hegerl et al., 2009). These programs include a broad array of components that target public opinion and knowledge or recognition of suicide, but also include a strong focus on improving access to and quality of mental health care within their health systems. An example is Maryland's youth suicide-prevention plan, which includes school programs, a state hotline, an acquired immune deficiency syndrome (AIDS) hotline, media education, and gun control (Goldsmith et al., 2002). Internationally, Finland, Australia, and England provide similar examples.

Another integrated approach is the suicide-prevention program in the Air Force, which demonstrated a reduction in suicides following implementation (Knox et al., 2003). The key element of the Air Force program was seen as the attempt to shift the culture within the Air Force to make suicide prevention a community-wide responsibility rather than a medical problem. The program showed significant and sustained reduction in suicide rates (Knox et al., 2003; Litts et al., 1999). The program included 11 key components that focused on leadership involvement, professional military education and guidelines for commanders, community preventive services, education and training, policy changes, and a suicide event surveillance system. Some experts interviewed said that the success of the Air Force program could not necessarily be transferred to other groups, even within the military, because the Air Force culture is unique and the program was tailored specifically for it. However, its proponents said that the defining feature of this program was the painstaking process by which it was developed and tailored to the Air Force, and that the same process could be used to tailor a program to the other branches of the military (we discuss the details of the Air Force program in Chapter Four). A unique aspect of the program was providing means for counselors to maintain confidentiality of treatment for suicidal intent under certain circumstances.

Finally, some rural tribal suicide-prevention programs also fall into this category of integrated approaches and can include such elements as cultural enhancement, increased mental health services, use of natural helpers, school programs, and socioeconomic improvements (Goldsmith et al., 2002). In addition, money awarded to states, tribal governments, and college campuses to develop suicide-prevention programs under the Garrett Lee Smith Memorial Act (Pub. L. 108-355) will fund the adoption of integrated approaches to prevent suicide. These programs are new and have yet to be officially evaluated.

Thus, whereas there is some evidence for the impact of integrated approaches, there have been no studies that dismantle them to demonstrate which components are critical to their impact, and they therefore provide little guidance in developing new programs.

Implications for DoD

The Air Force suicide-prevention program could provide a model for the other services. Some experts think that the cultural shift achieved in the Air Force model would be more difficult in the other services.

Integrated programs that offer universal prevention (health promotion and skill building) as well as targeted interventions for high-risk individuals can address the broad spectrum of suicidal behaviors.

Conclusion

In conclusion, some promising practices emerge from the current civilian literature, but much remains unknown in terms of best practices. Only a handful of studies have shown meaningful reductions in actual suicide attempts or deaths by suicide, and the rest of the best-practice literature relies on suggestive data or expert opinion. Thus, efforts in suicide prevention will need to continue to monitor the emerging literature and newer promising approaches, such as those that capitalize on telehealth and the Internet, newly emerging treatments, and results from evaluations of existing ones. Table 3.2 highlights the strength of evidence at present across the continuum of prevention programs.

From this table, we can derive six broad goals of a comprehensive suicide-prevention strategy:

1. *Raise awareness and promote self-care.* Reducing known risk factors, such as substance abuse and mental health problems, are often included as one aspect of integrated approaches. These efforts can be seen as part of suicide-prevention planning. One clear finding that emerges from the literature is that a focus on skill building may be important at all stages of prevention. This is a clear recommendation for universal prevention programs but is also supported by examination of the specific interventions that have been proven to work for reduction of suicide attempts. For those who have attempted suicide, programs with demonstrated success all use skill building to some degree, whether to build skills in stopping automatic thoughts that can lead to a suicidal crisis state, or whether teaching problem solving and more-effective ways of gaining social support.

2. *Identify those at high risk.* Suicide is an extremely rare phenomenon but is more frequent among certain groups, such as those with mental disorders or those who have recently experienced a negative life event. Selective and indicated prevention is a fundamental component of a public health approach to disease prevention and is predicated upon identifying those at higher risk. Thus, a comprehensive suicide-prevention program should have means by which this may occur, such as screening in primary care or through the use of gatekeepers.

3. *Facilitate access to quality care.* For someone who has been identified as being at increased risk for suicide, the evidence largely favors prevention programs based on a relationship between individuals and behavioral health-care providers. Past research highlights a number of barriers to behavioral health care in both the general population (Kessler, Berglund, et al., 2001) and some that are specific to the military (Schell and Marshall, 2008) (see Table 3.1 for commonly cited barriers to mental health treatment). Although reducing barriers to behavioral health care has not been specifically correlated with reducing suicides except as

Table 3.2
State of the Evidence Across Multiple Initiatives to Prevent Suicide

Program Type	Strongest Evidence	Mixed Evidence	Promising Approaches That Warrant Evaluation	Not Recommended but Commonly Used
Universal prevention				
School-based prevention programs that include skill building	x			
Prevention programs that raise awareness only, or short, didactic programs without follow-up				x
Selected or indicated prevention				
Physician training to detect depression and assess suicide risk	x			
Use of effective treatments for depression and other mental health problems, such as those found within primary-care collaborative care models	x			
DBT or CT for suicide attempters	x			
Integrated approaches across whole communities that combine several elements	x			
Caring letters or other outreach in the postcrisis period for suicide attempters or severely depressed individuals		x		
Assessment and crisis-management techniques, such as CAMS and SAFE VET			x	
No-suicide contracts used alone for crisis intervention				x
Inpatient hospitalization that does not include evidence-based treatments				x
Means restriction	x			
Postvention and media awareness			x	

part of broad, integrated programs, facilitating access to effective care will inevitably involve reducing these barriers.

4. *Provide quality care.* The need to ensure quality of mental health services is a critical and often-overlooked component of suicide prevention. Among the experts interviewed, some believed that a specific focus on suicidal behavior is key, using specialized techniques as found in DBT and CT for suicide. However, other experts believed that a general focus on mental health problems and a focus on relieving depression and anxiety would be sufficient to improve prevention of suicide. This tension between specialization for suicide and a more general focus on mental health has not been resolved and is highly relevant to how resources are allocated in suicide-prevention efforts. The VA's Blue Ribbon Work Group puts suicide prevention in the broader framework of comprehensive surveillance, research, and program evaluation for mental health, as well as specifying specific education, training, and quality improvement (QI) around suicide and use of SPCs.

5. *Restrict access to lethal means.* There is evidence that restricting access to lethal means is an effective way to prevent suicide, including the use of gun locks. This might be difficult in the U.S. military, due to the facts that (1) firearms are the most common means by which servicemembers kill themselves; (2) access to and use of firearms is a critical component of many servicemembers' jobs; and (3) in the United States, the Constitution preserves individuals' right to keep and bear arms, though gun laws vary across states by legal jurisdiction (Brady Campaign to Prevent Gun Violence, undated). However, programs in the VHA that attempt to improve safety of firearms, through the use of gun locks for veterans with children at home, for example, appear promising (Roeder et al., 2009).

6. *Respond appropriately to suicides and suicide attempts.* Given evidence of possible imitative suicides, suicide-prevention programs must have in place a strategy for responding to a completed suicide. Responding appropriately to the aftermath of a suicide death balances expressions of sympathy and understanding while not glorifying the decedent. Such a strategy should be focused on how details of the suicide are communicated in the media as well as how the information is passed on to groups to which the deceased individual belonged (e.g., classmates, colleagues, military unit).

These six tenets should be present across the entire mix of services for psychological health and safety promoted by NIMH (Schoenbaum, Heinssen, and Pearson, 2009). For example, proper self-care will reduce risk and promote skills in a universal program or by means of outpatient psychiatric services for those at risk. Similarly, identifying those at high risk for suicide and facilitating access to care are tasks important for gatekeepers as well as those who offer outpatient psychiatric services. Providing quality care is relevant to all who are responsible for dealing with persons who may be suicidal, including clergy as well as primary-care physicians and licensed psychiatrists and psychologists.

One issue that is not addressed at all in the review of best practices is the overlap in the military between the health-care and personnel systems. Most civilian research has focused on health care exclusively, without consideration of work or job performance issues, but the two are entwined in the military context. Experts we interviewed discussed issues relating to whether suicidal individuals should be kept in the treatment system after evaluation for suicide risk or whether they should be returned to the unit for "unit watch," for instance. In addition, current personnel policies do not provide information about the career ramifications of being labeled as a suicide risk or of getting mental health treatment or a mental health diagnosis, which can create uncertainty and reluctance among gatekeepers to bring attention to a peer in need. These types of issues that are unique to the military context are not addressed at all in the best-practice literature, and, therefore, there are really no data that can guide those policies and decisions.

CHAPTER FOUR
Suicide Prevention in the Department of Defense

In this chapter, we provide detailed information about the programs and initiatives that aim to prevent suicides in DoD and for each service in turn: the Army, Navy, Air Force, and Marine Corps. We begin our description of each service's suicide-prevention activities with what we find to be the overarching philosophy guiding suicide-prevention programs in that service. Following this, we provide an overview of the programs and initiatives each service has in place to prevent suicide, categorized as primary or universal prevention programs, selected or indicated prevention programs, and, finally, postvention programs and initiatives. We include programs offered specially to military personnel returning from deployment as selected or indicated prevention programs due to the increased risk these individuals have of developing mental health problems (described in Chapter Two). No service identified means-restriction policies as a component of its suicide-prevention program. The next chapter describes the support for suicide-prevention activities in each service with specific attention to the official documentation and organizations that support suicide prevention as well as how such activities are funded.

Our service-specific descriptions across these domains derive from the literature reviews and expert interviews we conducted. When possible, we attempted to provide the same level of detail for each service. However, this was not always possible, as the level of information available about suicide-prevention activities varies from service to service. We also include appendixes at the end of the monograph that describe in detail the specific programs and initiatives each service has in place to prevent suicide.

Department of Defense Initiatives

Five initiatives reach across all services that have bearing on suicide prevention in DoD.

First, SPARRC is composed of key stakeholders in preventing suicide from each service and from DoD, including each service's SPPM and representatives from the National Guard Bureau, Reserve Affairs, OAFME, National Center for Telehealth and Technology (T2), as well as representatives from the VA. The committee meets monthly and works to develop standard suicide reporting, rate calculations, and nomenclature;

to collaborate on an annual military suicide-prevention conference (described later); and to develop joint products and share best practices and program resources (Sutton, 2009).

Beginning in 2008, the Defense Centers of Excellence for Psychological Health and Traumatic Brain Injury (DCoE) began funding the Real Warriors Campaign, a public education initiative to address the stigma of seeking psychological care and treatment. To accomplish this goal, the campaign has produced public service announcements, social marketing materials on the campaign (e.g., fact sheet, press releases), and a public website with links to resources for active duty, Guard and reserve, veterans, families, and health professionals (DCoE, undated). Campaign ads and posters that are service specific are available for download on the website. As of February 2010, the campaign had also established collaborative relationships with 15 national, federal, and military organizations (e.g., National Military Family Association, Army Wounded Warrior Program), as well as five of DCoE's component centers (Center for the Study of Traumatic Stress, Center for Deployment Psychology, Deployment Health Clinical Center, Defense and Veterans Brain Injury Center, T2).

In 2009, DoD established a congressionally directed Department of Defense Task Force on the Prevention of Suicide by Members of the Armed Forces. The goals of the task force are to identify suicide trends and common causal factors, identify methods to establish or update suicide-prevention and education programs based on trends or common causal factors, assess each service's suicide-prevention and education programs, assess suicide incidence by military occupation, and assess multiple issues related to investigating suicides among military personnel. Findings from the task force are expected in the summer or fall of 2010 (Embrey, 2009a; DoD, 2009a).

Prior to 2008, each service had its own approach to suicide surveillance (e.g., ASER in the Army; Department of the Navy Suicide Incident Report [DONSIR] in the Navy; Suicide Event Surveillance System in the Air Force). As of January 1, 2008, each service now uses the DoDSER for required reporting of suspected suicide deaths and suicide attempts. The DoDSER is a form that contains approximately 250 data fields (e.g., demographics, military history) and must be completed for all suspected suicides and suicide attempts that result in hospitalization or evacuation, although, through the course of our key informant interviews, we were informed that each service has established different criteria for nonfatal suicidal behaviors. The DoDSER is managed by T2.

Since 2002, DoD has held a suicide-prevention conference. It is now organized by SPARRC and is attended by each service's SPPM as well as professional health-care consultants, counselors, chaplains, unit suicide-prevention officers, substance-abuse professionals, and unit leaders. It is designed as an opportunity for members of DoD to learn about innovative suicide-prevention and treatment programs. Beginning in 2009, the conference was held jointly across DoD and the VA.

Suicide Prevention in the Army

Philosophy of the Current Approach

In response to rising suicides among its population, the Army has initiated activities with the goal of increasing the emotional well-being of the force. There are two dominant themes for suicide prevention in recent times.

First, the Army's strategy for suicide prevention is based on the buddy system: "soldiers taking care of soldiers."[1] This is manifested foremost in recent training and awareness campaigns within the ACE program, which is predicated on peers playing an active role in encouraging and facilitating seeking help from services provided by the military and elsewhere.

Second, following recent increases in suicide-prevention activities, there has been a concerted effort to develop a more holistic view of mental health preparedness. In the case of the Deputy Chief of Staff for Army Operations (G-3)–run program Comprehensive Soldier Fitness (CSF), the effort is to look across five dimensions of strength—physical, emotional, social, family, and spiritual—to create more-resilient soldiers.[2] Suicide prevention is an outgrowth of the resilience that this program is attempting to foster within the entire force.

In recent years, the Army has also initiated multiple task forces and working groups and bolstered efforts to address concerns over escalating suicides within the military. In 2006, the Deputy Chief of Staff for Army Personnel (G-1) formed a working group to better integrate and synchronize efforts from various agencies, identify trends, and provide recommendations to senior Army leaders. In theater, a Multi-National Force—Iraq (MNF-I) task force was also formed to review trends and allocate resources as needed. In early 2009, the Army also stood up the interim ASPTF to provide immediate, coordinated reporting and programmatic solutions to reduce suicides within its ranks. The Army also increased the number of behavioral health-care providers, including increasing behavioral health personnel for units that have been in theater for more than six months and, since 2007, has increased the number of SPCs in the Active Component, the Army National Guard, and the U.S. Army Reserve.

Description of Programs and Initiatives

Primary Prevention: *Communication and Outreach.* The Army uses the Internet to convey information about suicide prevention. The Army Suicide Prevention Program (ASPP) website contains a number of links to information about suicide-prevention training and activities in the Army, including training briefings (discussed later),

---

[1]   The ASPTF states explicitly that the second enduring suicide-prevention message is "Suicide prevention is about Soldiers taking care of Soldiers" (Chiarelli, 2009, p. C-3).

[2]   See U.S. Army (undated) for more information on the CSF efforts within the Army.

videos, information papers, and links to other organizations and material (Deputy Chief of Staff, 2010).

The videos and presentations contained on the ASPP website fall under the guise of vignettes, scenarios, and training curricula for soldiers and leaders. The suicide-prevention training scenarios presentation (U.S. Department of the Army, 2008c) portrays 12 scenarios along with tactical, operational, and strategic questions and answers concerning each.[3] The scenarios cover the following broad topics: predeployment (three scenarios); warrior in transition; deployed female; postdeployment (two scenarios); deployed captain; deployed female staff sergeant; rest and relaxation; basic training; and deployed private first class (U.S. Department of the Army, 2008c). It is unclear how these topics were chosen.

The Army G-1 site also includes four videos called "Suicide Prevention Vignettes" under the title of "U.S. Armed Forces: Courage to Care."[4] The videos are listed in Table 4.1 along with short descriptions. The videos portray individuals in civilian clothes confessing to a camera about aspects of suicides.

The ASPP site also contains videos addressing specific aspects of suicides. For instance, a 16-minute video, "Soldiers, Stress, and Depression: Profiles in Personal Courage," contextualizes military suicide in the broader area of behavioral health through discussions with medical professionals and military personnel. It also contains some short vignettes of soldiers in situations to further illustrate the points. The video was originally produced by Command Surgeon's Office, U.S. Army Training

Table 4.1
Descriptions of Videos Available from the Army Suicide Prevention Program Website

Name	Time (min:sec)	Description
"Best Friend"	1:08	Individuals in a heightened emotional state describe the aftermath of a friend or colleague's suicide.
"Graveyard"	1:02	A lone friend or family member at a graveyard bemoans a suicide.
"Suicide Situation"	1:44	Individuals confess their feelings of responsibility for not caring for a friend in need of help.
"Warning Signs"	1:48	Individuals discuss their emotional state of mind consistent with suicidal ideation and behaviors.

---

[3] See Deputy Chief of Staff (2009a) for additional information. Strategic questions include "What resources are available to you to help prepare your unit?" The strategic questions cover organizational and operational considerations in advance of problems that might be encountered. An example tactical question is this: "What should you do once the soldier states he is willing to do anything to avoid deployment?" These questions address real-time responses to specific situations. Operational questions fall in between in terms of scope and specificity.

[4] Videos are available from Deputy Chief of Staff (2009b).

and Doctrine Command (TRADOC), with a message from TRADOC's deputy commanding general for initial military training.

The Army G-1 suicide-prevention website also contains a number of what the Army previously referred to as "life lines" but now calls *crisis intervention resources*—phone numbers that military personnel can call to find more information on suicide and seek help. Some of the numbers are listed in Table 4.2. These numbers are used throughout Army health-promotion sites and include both military specific and general health and emergency sites.

Posters related to suicide prevention are generally produced by CHPPM. The CHPPM website (CHPPM, 2009) contains examples of suicide-prevention posters. The posters are available for download and use across the Army and other services.

Education and Training. Four education or training programs can be categorized as primary suicide-prevention programs in the Army. First, there are suicide awareness briefings for leaders and shorter briefings for soldiers developed under the ASPP.[5] These briefings summarize background material on suicide, highlight the ACE program, present vignettes for discussion on suicide, and provide recommendations that leaders (or soldiers) can implement to reduce suicides. The leadership briefing, given by the commanding general or unit's sergeant major, focuses on actions leaders might take to establish a "command climate" conducive to soldiers seeking help. The soldier briefing, on the other hand, acknowledges the stresses that soldiers are likely feeling and provides information on resources available and encouragement for both self-care and caring for a peer who also may need help.

"Strong Bonds" is a chaplain-led initiative provided for military personnel who have previously deployed or who are about to deploy. It provides military couples,

Table 4.2
Crisis Intervention Resources Included on the Army Suicide Prevention Program Website

Name	Specific to Military?	Number
Army G-1, Army Well Being Liaison Office	Yes	1-800-833-6622
DCoE	Yes	1-866-966-1020
Emergency	No	911
Military OneSource Crisis Intervention Line	Yes	1-800-342-9647
Suicide Prevention Lifeline	No	1-800-273-TALK
Wounded Soldier and Family Hotline	Yes	1-800-984-8523

NOTE: This information was posted on the Army G-1 website as of March 30, 2010.

---

[5] Briefings are 25 slides (leaders) and 14 slides (soldiers) long and are available from Deputy Chief of Staff (2009b).

singles, and families the opportunity to interact with others who share similar deployment cycles, on voluntary weekend retreats. During these retreats, groups not only share their experiences but also learn about community resources that can help them in times of crisis.

Required suicide-prevention training was mandated on February 13, 2009, when Secretary of the Army Preston Geren ordered a stand-down in response to growing concern over suicides within the Army. As part of the stand-down, chain-teaching materials were provided to the troops. The stand-down is part of a three-phase response to suicides that unfolded during 2009, beginning with the release of the "Beyond the Front" interactive video. The interactive "Beyond the Front" video was created through a partnership between Lincoln University of Missouri and WILL Interactive using a behavior-modification technology known as a Virtual Experience Immersive Learning Simulation (VEILS®) (Sheftick, 2008). The video was distributed widely throughout the Army starting in early CY 2009. The second part of the three-part training is another video and supporting material called "Shoulder to Shoulder." The third phase is annual training utilizing existing suicide-prevention training resources.

Finally, the Army's new CSF program run out of G-3 includes among its planned initiatives Master Resiliency Trainers, who will be deployed to every battalion (Landstuhl Regional Medical Center Public Affairs, 2009). Although the CSF program does not currently state suicide prevention as a core activity, it is implied by the individual activities within its purview. Recent discussions with officials within the Army indicate that CSF will eventually include some suicide-prevention activities within its responsibilities.[6]

Selected or Indicated Prevention: *Gatekeeper Training.* The Army currently runs gatekeeper training programs that teach peers to act as gatekeepers, as well as a specific program for chaplains. The peer program was developed in response to an Army G-1 request that CHPPM develop a suicide intervention skill training support package (TSP) for Army-wide distribution (CHPPM, 2008). The result was CHPPM's ACE suicide intervention program.[7] It aims to teach soldiers how to recognize suicidal behavior in fellow soldiers and the warning signs that accompany it; target those sol-

---

[6] See U.S. Army (undated) for more information.

[7] The ACE program is similar to other past efforts. For instance, it resembles AID LIFE, a Navy and Marine Corps suicide awareness program. That acronym is short for *ask, intervene immediately, do not keep it a secret, locate help, inform the chain of command of the situation, find someone to stay with the person now,* and *expedite. Ask* means do not be afraid to ask, "Are you thinking about hurting yourself?" or "Are you thinking about suicide?" *Intervene immediately* urges the servicemember to take action and to listen and let the person know he or she is not alone. *Do not keep it a secret* is self-explanatory. *Locate help* means to seek out the officer on duty, chaplain, physician, corpsman, friend, family member, crisis-line worker, or emergency-room staff. *Inform the chain of command of the situation* is urged because the chain of command can secure necessary assistance resources for the long term. Suicide risk does not get better with quick solutions. Effective problem-solving takes time, and the chain of command can monitor progress to help avert future difficulties. *Find someone to stay with the person now* means simply not to leave the person alone. Finally, *expedite* means to get help now: An at-risk person needs immediate

diers most at risk for suicide and the least likely to seek help due to stigma; increase a soldier's confidence to ask whether a battle buddy is thinking of suicide; teach soldiers skills in active listening; and encourage soldiers to take a battle buddy directly to the chain of command, chaplain, or behavioral health provider. The ACE program includes training information using DVDs, briefings, handouts, and training tip cards (wallet cards) all readily accessible through the web, to increase a soldier's ability to find and help fellow soldiers at risk for suicide. The ACE program training is meant to take three hours and is designed to be administered at the platoon level (Cartwright, 2009).

Gatekeeper training is offered to chaplains and others to reinforce training at unit level under the ASIST activity (U.S. Army, undated). Under ASIST, the Army provides workshops and interactive CDs about how to provide help to those experiencing suicidal thoughts and those trying to help them. The training does not produce personnel qualified to diagnose mental disorders or directly treat individuals, but rather provides necessary training for first responders until a professional behavioral health specialist can be located. The Army's suicide-prevention policy is to have at least two ASIST-trained representatives per installation, camp, state, territory, and Reserve Support Center. In addition, all chaplains and their assistants, behavioral health professionals, and Army Community Service staff members must also attend the training (Maxwell, 2009). Since 2001, thousands of ASIST kits have been distributed within the Army (U.S. Army, undated).

Programs for Deployed Personnel. Personnel returning from deployment are offered specific programs that may prevent suicide among this cohort. Resiliency training is offered via the Army's resilience training (formerly Battlemind) program, which is a compendium of information provided to soldiers on the web in order "to prepare Warriors mentally for the rigors of combat and other military deployments" (U.S. Department of the Army, 2008b). The information is largely focused on what soldiers can expect to experience once deployed and how to transition once returned. Suicide prevention is not currently addressed directly in resilience training. As described in Chapter Two, returning military personnel are required to complete the PDHA administered to soldiers immediately upon return from theater, and the Post-Deployment Health Reassessment (PDHRA), which is administered 90–180 days after returning. Both assessments screen for PTSD and depression and ask specifically about suicide ideation. How these assessments are used remains unclear.

Postvention. In response to a suicide, each Army installation is required to have in place an Installation Suicide Response Team (ISRT). The ISRT is intended to offer support to unit commanders, including how to talk to the media about suicides.[8] The

---

attention from professional caregivers. See U.S. Navy (2005). The Navy's ACT campaign is also similar. More information on it can be found in the next section of this chapter and in Appendix B.

[8] ISRTs have recently been changed to Suicide Response Teams (SRTs), as of the most recent version of AR 600-63 (dated September 20, 2009).

Army also provides access through its websites to information from external organizations focused on reducing and coping with the aftermath of suicide, including a guide for those who plan memorial services and provide support to family members and friends, a booklet on coping with grief after a suicide, and a guide for financial decisionmaking after a spouse, parent, child, or loved one dies by suicide.

Suicide Prevention in the Navy

Philosophy of Current Initiatives

The Navy's approach to suicide prevention is guided by a philosophy that considers stress a key factor contributing to suicidal behavior. The Navy conceptualizes stress along a continuum, depicted in the Navy's stress continuum model visual aid (see Figure 4.1), which provides sailors, leaders, and family members a tool for assessing stress responses. It promotes the idea that, prior to experiencing a stressor, sailors should be "ready," which means that they are well-trained and in cohesive units and ready families. In the face of a stressor, the model indicates that sailors will react (e.g., may be anxious or have behavioral change), could become injured (e.g., persistent distress), or become ill (e.g., injuries that do not heal or get worse). It also indicates that caring for sailors across the continuum is the responsibility of unit leaders, individuals, shipmates, and families, as well as caregivers, with unit leaders assuming most of the responsibility in ensuring that their sailors are "ready" and caregivers assuming most of the responsibility when sailors are "ill."

Figure 4.1
Stress Injury Continuum

Ready (Green)	Reacting (Yellow)	Injured (Orange)	Ill (Red)
• Good to go • Well trained • Prepared • Fit and focused • Cohesive units and ready families	• Distress or impairment • Mild and transient • Anxious, irritable, or sad • Behavior change	• More severe or persistent distress or impairment • Leaves lasting memories, reactions, and expectations	• Stress injuries that don't heal without help • Symptoms persist for >60 days, get worse, or initially get better and then return worse
Unit-leader responsibility	Individual, shipmate, family responsibility		Caregiver responsibility

SOURCE: Adapted from MCCS (2007c).
RAND MG953-4.1

Interviewees indicated that the underlying philosophy of addressing stress problems early and facilitating access to caregivers (e.g., chaplains and behavioral healthcare providers at MTFs) also contribute to preventing suicide (Kraft and Westphal, undated). The Navy's approach to suicide prevention emphasizes early intervention for situations that may cause stressful reactions for sailors, such as relationship problems or financial troubles (Chavez, 2009a).

Description of Programs and Initiatives

Primary Prevention: *Communication and Outreach.* The NMCPHC and Navy Safety Center assist in communicating about suicide awareness to all sailors through leadership messages, newsletters, posters, brochures, videos, and other forums (Chavez, 2009b). The Navy has created a suite of four posters that target suicide prevention by advertising the ACT model and offer messages that sailors are not alone, one person can save a life, and sailors are "all in this together."[9] Two brochures were published in November 2008: a resource for suicide prevention and a summary of the stress continuum depicted in Figure 4.1.[10] There is also a 32-second public service announcement (PSA) that educates sailors about symptoms of suicidal behaviors and encourages sailors to inform command if they are concerned about a fellow sailor.[11]

In May 2009, the Operational Stress Control (OSC) program and the Personal Readiness and Community Support branch sponsored a short survey (the 2009 Behavioral Health Quick Poll) to assess perceptions of stress and suicide prevention among sailors (Newell, Whittam, and Uriell, 2009). The survey revealed the following:

- The majority of sailors have attended suicide-prevention training in the past year. Most training was provided either by a person within sailors' commands or via online modules, although respondents indicated that they preferred training by a person (e.g., Fleet and Family Support Center [FFSC] staff, medical staff) to online training.
- The majority of sailors believed that there would be negative consequences for a sailor who sought help for suicidal thoughts (e.g., the survey captured responses such as "command would treat person differently," "negative impact on career," and "not able to keep security clearance").
- Approximately half the officers and enlisted sailors know their command's SPC, and many know what to do if a fellow sailor talks about suicide.
- Sailors reported that their commands are taking action to prevent suicide.

---

[9]   Posters are available online for download from Navy Personnel Command (NAVPERS) (2009).

[10] Brochure is available for download online from NAVPERS (2009).

[11] The PSA is available online for download from NMCPHC (2009a).

Education and Training. The annual suicide-prevention awareness training is a General Military Training (GMT) given to all sailors and intended to provide them with the knowledge and action strategies needed to understand and recognize the signs and symptoms of potential suicidality in a peer.[12] The training utilizes a video different from the aforementioned PSA, "Making the Critical Decision." This video describes the role of a good sailor in preventing suicide, reviews suicidal thinking and key risk factors, includes a testimonial from a sailor, and walks through a dramatized example of how to intervene with a sailor exhibiting signs that he or she may be suicidal. At the time of this writing, Personal Readiness and Community Support Branch (OPNAV N135) and Naval Education and Training Command (NETC) were collaborating with the Navy Media Center (now Defense Media Activity) to develop a new video for suicide awareness training. The video is purported to include interviews with command and family members affected by suicides and sailors and family members who helped prevent suicides (Chavez, 2009a).

The Navy's OSC program is a training program designed to build the skills needed to cope with stress and improve the psychological health of sailors and their families. It leads the naval approach to suicide prevention. The program provides training and practical decisionmaking tools for sailors, leaders, caregivers, and families so they can build resilience, identify stress responses, and mitigate problem stress (NAVADMIN 182/07). Sailors receive training on how to identify when they are stressed, healthy coping styles, and how to help distressed peers cope with stress. Leaders receive training in stress management and how to assess stress levels among their sailors. Caregivers receive training on how to assess and treat stress injuries and illnesses and provide psychological first aid and self-care. Families receive training on how to identify when they or their servicemember is stressed and provide support for their children and spouse.

The OSC training aims to encourage sailors, families, caregivers, and leaders to proactively address stress reactions and injuries before they become stress-related illnesses, including suicidal behaviors. To achieve this aim, the OSC training teaches three core principles: (1) Recognize when shipmates are in trouble, (2) break the code of silence and ask shipmates about what is going on, and (3) connect shipmates to the next level of support in the chain of command (Westphal, 2008).

A guide for leaders was developed to support the training and provides information on how to recognize a sailor in distress and describes a broad range of supportive interventions, resources, and strategies for leaders to support such sailors. The OSC program has also produced handbooks for sailors, families, and commands of indi-

---

[12] The training material used for this GMT are available online for download from NMCPHC (2009a).

vidual augmentees,[13] training modules on combat stress, and handouts and posters on coping with stress and dealing with insomnia (NMCPHC, 2009b).

Command-Level Programs. Command-level suicide-prevention programs are directed at all sailors and consist of a written crisis response plan that any sailor on duty can use to access emergency contacts, phone guidance, and basic safety precautions to assist a sailor at acute risk. An SPC is also appointed for each command to ensure that the required program components are in place.[14] An interviewee commented that commanders need flexibility in how they implement suicide-prevention programs because sailors may be aboard aircraft carriers, submarines, at shore, or in theater.

Psychological health education (e.g., training on OSC, workshop for returning sailors to address deployment stress) is also offered to all reservists through the Psychological Health Outreach program (Torsch, undated). In this program, Psychological Health Outreach coordinators are located at each Naval Operational Support Center (NOSC) (i.e., centers are located in each state, and each houses a command ombudsman who serves as the point of contact, or POC, for reservists) and provide assessment and referral and coordinate care and follow-up for reservists receiving services from MTFs, clinics and hospitals run by the VHA, and civilian providers. To monitor implementation and success of the Psychological Health Outreach coordinator program, program staff reported during our interview that they were tracking and reporting annually on the number of people contacted through outreach, the number of people served as clients, and the number of cases closed.

Selected or Indicated Prevention: *Gatekeeper Training.* There are four programs aimed specifically at training gatekeepers, though participation in these programs is never mandatory. The front-line supervisors' training is an interactive half-day workshop designed to assist front-line leaders (petty officers and junior officers) to recognize and respond to sailors in distress. Front-line leaders are targeted for this initiative because they supervise and have direct contact with a large number of sailors (Chavez, 2009a). Personal readiness summits are optional professional development opportunities in which front-line leaders, first responders, and command-appointed SPCs can get information about the OSC program, alcohol- and drug-abuse prevention, physical readiness, and sexual-assault prevention. The summits are supplemented by breakout sessions on specific topic areas, including suicide prevention. During personal readiness summits, trainers administer pre- and posttest questionnaires to assess whether trainees are familiar with content and evaluate whether the course is increasing trainees' confidence level in helping sailors or marines in distress. Currently, the questionnaires are not standardized across training modules and, at the time of this writing, had not yet been analyzed. The third training, the first responders' seminar, teaches

---

[13] An individual augmentee is a sailor who is being deployed as an individual instead of with a ship, squadron, or battalion.

[14] A checklist for command-level suicide-prevention programs is available online from NAVPERS (2010a).

first responders how to handle a sailor in crisis. Finally, gatekeepers can also receive information about suicide prevention at annual fleet suicide-prevention conferences (Chavez, 2009a).

Programs for Caregivers. The OSC program trains caregivers (typically chaplains, social workers, psychiatric technicians, and command leaders) about potential stress injuries associated with their professional responsibilities and the importance of developing and following a self-care plan (Westphal, 2008). The caregiver OSC training is being evaluated by the Center for Naval Analyses and was planned to be completed in December 2009 (though, as of March 2010, there were still no results). The evaluation assesses how caregivers' work-related stress affects patient safety over time.

Programs for Deployed Personnel. The Returning Warriors Workshops (RWWs) are voluntary weekend retreats during which chaplains and counselors provide additional support to sailors returning from deployment and their spouses. The workshops are designed to help ameliorate feelings of stress, isolation, and other psychological and physical disorders and injuries, especially PTSD and TBI (Torsch, undated). Program staff for the RWWs were also tracking and reporting annually on the number of sailors and spouses who attend RWWs, results from workshop evaluations to measure participant satisfaction, and results from after-action reports that highlight challenges to program implementation and participation and action plans to resolve the challenges.

Postvention. There are currently no initiatives directed at postvention. However, three groups of individuals within the naval personnel system can assist families and units that have lost a member to suicide. Casualty assistance calls officers (CACOs) serve as the Navy's official representatives to assist family members of active-duty sailors who have died, are missing, or are seriously ill or very seriously injured. CACOs provide family members with information about the circumstances of the sailor's death, help families with immediate needs, and provide assistance in making funeral or memorial arrangements as appropriate. Additionally, CACOs assist the family and any other beneficiaries in the preparation and submission of claims to various government agencies for benefits to which they may be entitled (NAVPERS, undated). Chaplains also provide support to families and units and provide counseling and assistance with memorial services. Finally, upon request, Special Psychiatric Rapid Intervention Teams (SPRINTs) are available to assist commands by providing debriefings and emotional support to a unit following a traumatic event, including a unit member's suicide. SPRINT teams are located on each coast (Norfolk and San Diego). Local installation response teams also provide services similar to SPRINT teams (Chavez, 2009a).

Suicide Prevention in the Air Force

Philosophy of Current Initiatives

Senior Air Force leadership resolved to formally address the problem of suicide in the Air Force in 1996 following the suicide of Navy Admiral Jeremy Boorda and an increasing number of suicides among active-duty Air Force personnel. In 1996, the Air Force Vice Chief of Staff commissioned the Air Force Suicide Prevention Integrated Product Team (IPT). The team was instructed to develop a comprehensive plan to respond to the increasing number of suicides among active-duty Air Force personnel. It did so by reviewing all available information about Air Force personnel who died by suicide, holding briefings on available suicide data, reviewing suicide theories, and meeting regularly to discuss Air Force policy and culture. From this process, the IPT determined that many suicides in the Air Force are preventable and that suicide was a problem of the entire Air Force community. Thus, it determined that a community approach to preventing suicide headed by the Air Force Chief of Staff (AF/CC) and four-star generals would be the most effective means to reach all Air Force members and encourage and protect those who responsibly seek mental health treatment (AFPAM 44-160).

The IPT developed a suicide-prevention program that consists of 11 initiatives for base-level suicide-prevention programs:

1. Leadership Involvement
2. Addressing Suicide Prevention Through Professional Military Education
3. Guidelines for Commanders: Use of Mental Health Services
4. Community Preventive Services
5. Community Education and Training
6. Investigative Interview Policy
7. Traumatic Stress Response (TSR)
8. Integrated Delivery System (IDS) and Community Action Information Board (CAIB)
9. Limited Privilege Suicide Prevention (LPSP) Program
10. IDS Consultation Assessment Tool
11. Suicide Event Surveillance System (SESS) (AFPAM 44-160).

Prior to 2008, one of the 11 tenets was Monitoring the Air Force Suicide Prevention Program (AFSPP). This was done through the SESS, in which data on all Air Force active-duty suicides and suicide attempts were entered into a central database in order to track suicide events and facilitate identification of potential risk factors for suicide in Air Force personnel (AFPAM 44-160). As of 2008, the SESS is being fully replaced by the DoDSER. In addition, an AFSPP checklist was developed to facilitate monitoring the implementation of the 11 initiatives of the AFSPP. The checklist is completed for each installation and signed by the IDS chair, the CAIB executive director, and the CAIB chair.

As described in Chapter Three, the Air Force program takes an integrated approach to preventing suicides that has been associated with a 33-percent risk reduction for suicide in the six years since the program was implemented, relative to the six years prior (Knox et al., 2003). It has been reviewed by the Substance Abuse and Mental Health Services Administration's National Registry of Evidence-Based Programs and Practices, which found that the research strategy was strong enough to support the claimed decreases in relative risk of suicide (see SAMHSA, 2010). Many suicide-prevention programs outside of the military have been modeled after the Air Force program. It is also described in Appendix C.

Description of Programs and Initiatives

Primary Prevention: *Leadership Involvement.* This initiative requires that the AF/CC, other senior leaders, and base commanders actively support the suicide-prevention initiatives in the Air Force community by communicating with its members and fully engaging in suicide-prevention efforts (AFPAM 44-160). The AF/CC disseminates information about the suicide-prevention program in order to ensure that all commanders and personnel receive it in a timely manner and to emphasize the priority and importance of the information.

Education and Training. Two initiatives involve training and education in suicide prevention. First, suicide prevention is incorporated into all formal military training (i.e., addressing suicide prevention through professional military education). The IPT established learning outcomes for each of the three levels of enlisted professional military education, as well as the three levels of officer professional military education and the First Sergeant Academy. The suicide-prevention element of all professional military education includes background knowledge about suicide (such as warning signs and implications of seeking treatment), personal coping skills (such as problem-solving and conflict resolution), peer support skills (such as knowing what to say and where to get help), and leadership skills (such as prevention steps that commanders should take) (AFPAM 44-160).

In addition, all military and civilian employees in the Air Force receive annual suicide-prevention training on risk factors for suicide, intervention skills, and referral procedures for those at risk. This training is described in Air Force instruction (AFI) 44-154, Suicide and Violence Prevention Education and Training, and training materials are available on the AFSPP website (U.S. Air Force, undated). The program is adapted from the Air Education and Training Command LINK (look for possible concerns, inquire about concerns, note level of risk, and know referral resources and strategies) suicide-prevention program; its goal is to improve early identification and referral of those who are potentially at risk in order to prevent suicide, other self-defeating behavior, or behavior that may put others at risk. To reach this goal, the program focuses on decreasing stigma associated with seeking help, promoting early identification and referral of at-risk individuals by friends and coworkers, and encouraging supervisors to act as gateways to helping resources. In 1999, the IPT revised the training requirements so that they would focus on two levels of intervention: nonsupervisory "buddy care" training and leadership or supervisory training (AFPAM 44-160). The training modules are updated as needed. At the time of this writing, the Air Force has adopted the Army's ACE program, and interactive video clips have been integrated into the computer-based training. Additional training videos, including a "Message Home" video and discussion guide, are available on the AFSPP website (U.S. Air Force, undated).

Command-Level Programs. At each installation, an IDS organizes and coordinates overlapping prevention missions of participating agencies (chaplains, child and youth programs, Family Advocacy, Family Support, Health Promotion/Health and Wellness Centers, and outpatient mental health clinics [formerly Life Skills Support Centers], which provide individual therapy and counseling, stress- and anger-management programs, substance-abuse counseling, and other programs) while maintaining each organization's individual mission (AFPAM 44-160). Its purpose is to develop a comprehensive and coordinated plan for integrating community outreach and prevention programs, including suicide prevention, and to eliminate duplication, overlap, and gaps in delivering prevention services by consolidating existing committees with similar charters (AFI 90-501). The IDS provides centralized information and referral, assesses risk factors at the community and unit levels, and delivers prevention services and collaborative marketing of its information and referral preventive services.

The IDS is a standing subcommittee of the installation-level CAIB. At each installation, the CAIB was established to provide oversight and continuing guidance for implementation of the IDS and formal management structure of the AFSPP outside of the suicide-prevention IPT. The installation-level CAIB acquires information from the community through focus groups, surveys, town meetings, and interviews in order to identify issues related to individuals, families, and the community. Its members devise solutions to cross-organizational problems that cannot be addressed by individual CAIB organizations.

There are also CAIBs at each major command (MAJCOM) and at Air Force Headquarters. The MAJCOM CAIB reviews concerns that cannot be addressed at the installation level, organizes resources to be utilized for cross-organizational activities to promote quality of life in the Air Force community, and identifies community issues and recommendations for the CAIB at Air Force Headquarters. The Air Force Headquarters CAIB reviews issues that cannot be addressed by leadership at the MAJCOM or installation level and makes policy recommendations to Air Force or DoD leadership.

CAIBs at each level review the results of the Air Force community needs assessments and other quality-of-life surveys, address implications of the results, and formulate action items to address them. Each level is also required to prepare a Community Capacity Action Plan every two years to direct the CAIB's activities and determine priorities for the organizations participating in the CAIB.

In 2004, commands were encouraged to review and reenergize their CAIBs in order to ensure that they were meeting the needs of wing and MAJCOM installations (R. Brown, 2004).

Another command-level initiative provides commanders the opportunity to request an IDS Consultation Assessment Tool to assess unit strengths and identification of areas of vulnerability. The assessment provides information about behavioral health factors, such as alcohol-use frequency, emotional distress, lack of cooperation with partner, psychological distress, and job dissatisfaction. The commander can use results from this tool, with assistance from IDS consultants, to design interventions to support the health and welfare of his or her personnel (AFPAM 44-160).

Community prevention efforts (community education based on AFI 44-154, consulting, and outreach activities) are designed to reach those who are in need of services but do not seek individual treatment. At each installation, community-level personnel are intended to provide nonstigmatized alternatives to traditional behavioral health care, with the hope that these personnel will allow for earlier access to those at risk of suicide and provide preventive and educational services without the recordkeeping that discourages individuals from seeking help. The IPT recommended adding personnel to each base to carry out these preventive services; however, a change in the manpower standard allowed these preventive services to be provided by existing behavioral health personnel, such as psychologists and counselors working at outpatient mental health clinics, through the base-level IDS. Time spent in preventive activities was tracked through the Medical Expense and Performance Reporting System (MEPRS). In 1998, mental health personnel tripled the amount of time spent on prevention, and this amount remained steady through 1999; however, this time spent did not meet the goal of allotting 5 percent of all mental health activities to prevention (AFPAM 44-160).

Selected or Indicated Prevention: *Gatekeeper Training.* Commanders receive guidance (in the form of a briefing with a cover letter from the AF/CC) on the appropriate methods and situations for using mental health services and information about their role in encouraging early help-seeking behavior (AFPAM 44-160). This includes examples of circumstances that warrant referral to behavioral health-care providers, such as problems with alcohol, the law, finances, job performance, and relationships. Referral types and options, as well as implications of commander-directed referral, are discussed. The Leader's Guide for Managing Personnel in Distress and Leaders Suicide Prevention Briefings are available on the AFSPP website (U.S. Air Force, undated).

In 2008, the AFSPP released its Frontline Supervisors Training (FST), a voluntary half-day interactive workshop for units and individual supervisors (Loftus, 2008a). The basic message of the course is built around the acronym PRESS (prepare, recognize, engage, send, sustain). The course builds on skills that were taught as part of annual suicide-prevention training and professional military education and focuses on supervisory skills to help front-line supervisors recognize and assist those who are at risk of suicide or in need of behavioral health services (U.S. Department of the Air Force, undated).

Similar to that in the Army, gatekeeper training is offered to Air Force chaplains under ASIST, described in more detail under the discussion of the Army's gatekeeper training programs earlier in this chapter. We were informed that all Air Force chaplains have been trained in ASIST.

Policies and Procedures. The AFSPP determined the period following an arrest or investigative interview to be a high-risk time for suicide. The investigative-interview policy requires that, after any investigative interview, the investigator notify the airman's commander, first sergeant, or supervisor through person-to-person contact that the airman was interviewed and notified that he or she was under investigation and that those appearing emotionally distraught after an interview will be released only to their commander, first sergeant, supervisor, or appointed designee after any investigative interview (Jumper, 2002b; AFPAM 44-160). It then becomes the unit representative's responsibility to assess the individual's emotional state and contact a behavioral health provider if there is an indication of suicidal thoughts. Agencies without legal rights to detain an individual must make reasonable efforts to "hand off" the individual to a member of his or her unit or make notification as soon as possible if a hand-off is not feasible. If the unit leader determines that the individual is at risk for suicide, he or she is required to accompany the individual to a helping agency for professional care. Pamphlets about this initiative are available on the AFSPP website (U.S. Air Force, undated).

Due to the nature of military operations, confidentiality of servicemembers is not always protected (Burnam et al., 2008). Communications between a patient and behavioral health-care provider are kept confidential unless there is a legitimate need to disclose that information, such as when the behavioral health-care provider believes that the individual may be a danger to him or herself (AFI 44-109). The perceived access to servicemembers' medical and personal information by commanders and concerns about mental health records affecting one's career compounds the stigma and reluctance to seek mental health care and services. To encourage those who need mental health services to seek help, especially those who need it during times of disciplinary action, the IPT developed the LPSP program, which is described in AFI 44-109, Mental Health, Confidentiality, and Military Law (see also AFPAM 44-160). The program applies to members with charges who have been referred in a court martial or after notification of intent to impose punishment under Article 15 or Article 30 of the Uniform Code of Military Justice (UCMJ). The LPSP indicates that, for those in the program, information revealed to a behavioral health-care provider may not be utilized in the UCMJ action and cannot be used to characterize service at time of separation. Individuals are eligible for the LPSP program from the time of official notification that they are under investigation. Commanders place members in the program when they recognize that the individual may be at risk for suicide and have consulted with a behavioral health professional. The privilege is sustained until the member is no longer suicidal. Commanders may be notified of communications between a patient and psychotherapist for administrative purposes under law, AFI 44-109, and other instructions (such as the nuclear personnel reliability program or concern about danger to person or property).

Programs for Caregivers. Although not a tenet of the official AFSPP, in 2005, the Air Force published the Air Force Guide for Managing Suicidal Behavior (AFMOA, undated), which includes not only information for behavioral health-care providers but also recommendations for screening high-risk patients for suicidality in primary-care settings (Oordt et al., 2005). In 2007, staff at the SPRC visited Air Force bases across the country to offer a one-time training in assessment and management of suicidal behavior for mental health clinical staff (psychologists, psychiatrists, and social workers). Mental health providers trained in the Air Force's internships and residency programs receive training from providers who have already been trained, and training materials (e.g., a manual, training videos, and assessment measures) are provided to each clinic for those who have not received the training. In addition, documentation of risk assessments and utilization of procedures specified for high-risk/high-interest patients are monitored as part of the Air Force's Health Services Inspections.

Programs for Deployed Personnel. The Landing Gear program serves as a standardized preexposure preparation training program for deploying airmen, as well as the behavioral health component of reintegration education for returning airmen (Pflanz, 2008). The program addresses several behavioral health concerns (e.g., PTSD, depression, substance abuse, deployment stress) and refers to the Air Force's other programs for suicide prevention. During the predeployment training, airmen learn about deployment stress, the deployed environment, typical reactions, reintegration and reunion, prevention, and getting help. The postdeployment training focuses on the same topics as the predeployment training but emphasizes typical reactions, reintegration and reunion, and getting help. Behavioral health personnel or qualified IDS members typically deliver the briefing, and the trainings are provided as a freestanding class or in conjunction with other briefings provided by the Airman and Family Readiness Center and chaplains. The installation determines the frequency and scheduling of classes. Base commanders and behavioral health personnel determine who should receive the predeployment training, and, although it is recommended for all airmen, especially those deploying from high-risk groups, it is not required.

Postvention. Of the AFSPP's 11 initiatives, one is specifically geared to postvention. TSR (formerly Critical Incident Stress Management) teams were created to respond to traumatic incidents (e.g., terrorist attacks, serious accidents, suicide). The teams assist Air Force personnel in confronting their reactions to traumatic incidents (AFPAM 44-160). The IPT assisted in developing AFI 44-153, Traumatic Stress

Response, as a guideline for the Air Force response to traumatic events (AFI 44-153). The instruction requires that trained, multidisciplinary teams at each installation respond to local traumatic events. Consisting of behavioral health-care providers, medical providers, chaplains, and senior noncommissioned officers (NCOs) in nonmedical positions, these teams are structured to reduce the impression that counseling after trauma is only for those who need to see a behavioral health-care provider; broaden the skills, perspectives, and expertise delivered to participants; and reduce the impact on any one unit responding to a traumatic event.

A memorandum from the AF/CC supported this initiative, stating that each MAJCOM should have a postsuicide assessment process available and in place (Jumper, 2002a). Guidelines for such a process are available, but commands were encouraged to create or modify a process that best fits their individual community. In the event of a death by suicide, the process should include a protocol that would allow the command to share lessons learned from the event with the entire Air Force.

Suicide Prevention in the Marine Corps

Philosophy of Current Initiatives

The USMC uses a community approach to suicide prevention, as detailed in the Personal Services Manual (MCO P1700.24B). The Marine Corps relies primarily on gatekeeper programs in which local commands and front-line leaders, as well as the marines themselves, are trained to identify and refer those at risk for suicide to the appropriate resources (e.g., a commander, chaplain, behavioral health professional). This manual suggests that suicides often occur in association with problems that can be treated, such as relationship problems, alcohol abuse, and depression. Therefore, the manual purports that early identification of and intervention with marines exhibiting problem behavior will reduce the likelihood that these issues will detract from personal and unit readiness or lead to suicidal behavior.

Description of Programs and Initiatives

Primary Prevention: *Communication and Outreach.* Public information on suicide prevention is communicated through a variety of media, much of which is contained on the Marine Corps suicide-prevention website (MCCS, 2007a). These include a poster that presents military and national suicide statistics and resources for marines in distress, a suicide-prevention brochure, and videos that address the signs and symptoms of suicide and can be viewed online or on DVD, by request (see Table 4.3). In addition, the Marine Corps Suicide Prevention Program (MCSPP) sent all installations a copy of a play written and performed by marines and a video that showed a 40-minute performance of the play, which was a drama on suicide prevention. At the

Table 4.3
Marine Corps Suicide-Prevention Videos

Name	Time (min:sec)	Brief Description
Good Charlotte video	5:06	Music video for song "Hold On"; stories of suicide survivors are included at the beginning of the video, and suicide-prevention resources are referenced at the end of the video
"Got It Covered: Story of a Marine Unit"	4:19	Presents a vignette of a marine at risk for suicide and describes the warning signs and potential actions for intervening with a marine at risk for suicide
"Suicide Awareness: Making the Critical Decision"	14:56	Educational video that describes the risk factors and warning signs associated with suicide and provides guidance about when to intervene with a marine in distress
"You Are Not Alone"	3:33	Short video that briefly reviews signs and symptoms of suicide and includes a section in which marines share their experiences intervening with suicide

time of this writing, we were also told that six new posters were being developed but were not yet available for distribution.

Specific web-based resources are also available on the suicide-prevention website, including the Leaders Guide for Managing Marines in Distress; links for online classes in which chaplains, medical, and behavioral health-care providers can earn continuing education units; suicide-prevention briefing materials; resource guides for chaplains, medical, and mental health providers; and links to suicide-prevention hotlines and Military OneSource.

Finally, Combat Operational Stress Control (COSC) also produces informational materials to support its training and education efforts. For example, there is a Combat Operational Stress Decision Flowchart, which is a tool that marine leaders can use to help determine the level of functioning of their marines and family members (U.S. Marine Corps Forces Reserve, undated).

Education and Training. Suicide-prevention training is required for all new marines and offered as part of their required entry-level education. Enlisted marines and officers receive training in suicide awareness and prevention during boot camp and officer candidate and basic school. Additionally, drill instructors responsible for this entry-level education receive specialized training in suicide prevention. All marines also receive suicide awareness and prevention training during their mandatory martial-arts training using a module developed in 2008 by the Martial Arts Center of Excellence in Quantico in consultation with the Marine Corps SPPM. Additionally, interviewees indicated that the Marine Corps has required annual awareness training in suicide prevention since 1997.

Training and Education Command (TECOM) works with the MCSPP office to develop all training materials, including videos, briefings, and distance learning courses. These materials are supplemented at each installation with information on local procedures and resources. It is suggested that all commands provide such training annually, but local commands decide where and when to implement the training (MCO P1700.24B).

Through the Leadership Continuum training series, marines promoted from corporal to sergeant receive specific training designed to teach them the skills they will need to fulfill their new leadership position. Included in this training are a suicide-prevention module and a module on the stress continuum, described in the "Suicide Prevention in the Navy" section of this chapter.

Front-line leaders (i.e., NCOs and lieutenants) are offered voluntary training on suicide prevention through a front-line supervisors' training course taught by Marine Corps Semper Fit health-promotion personnel.[15] The front-line supervisors' training course was designed to teach these front-line leaders how to recognize and respond to marines in distress (Werbel, 2009). NCOs are also offered a specific peer-led training, "Never Leave a Marine Behind," which is organized around a video that includes interviews with spouses and marines who have been touched by suicide (Werbel, 2009). We were told that eight regional master training teams were taught by MCSPP staff to administer train-the-trainer courses, through which they then trained approximately 1,300 sergeant instructors in July and August 2009. By the end of October 2009, almost all of the approximately 70,000 NCOs in the Marine Corps were trained using the "Never Leave a Marine Behind" curriculum. The Uniformed Services University of the Health Sciences is currently evaluating the effectiveness of the course (Werbel, 2009).

COSC delivers programs at each installation to prevent, identify, and holistically treat mental injuries caused by combat or other operations. COSC programs include training to promote awareness of stress-related injuries and illness and to teach marines and their families the skills needed to understand and combat stress. The Marine Corps Operational Stress Surveillance and Training (MOSST) is a progression of educational briefs, health assessments, and leadership tools offered across the deployment cycle (i.e., predeployment, during deployment, immediately after deployment, three to six months postdeployment) designed to prevent, identify early, and manage operational stress at all levels (Gaskin and Feeks, 2007).

Command-Level Programs. Commands are asked to develop a suicide-prevention program that integrates and sustains awareness education, early identification and referral of at-risk personnel, treatment, and follow-up services. Annual suicide awareness training, postvention support, and reporting suicides using the DoDSER are also components of the Marine Corps command-level programs. The Marine Corps evaluates each command's suicide-prevention activities through the Commanding General Inspection Program and the Marine Corps Inspector General during every command inspection.

---

[15] Semper Fit is the sports, recreation, and fitness branch of the USMC.

Selected or Indicated Prevention: *Gatekeeper Training.* The "Are You Listening?" program is a two-day training for civilian staff affiliated with Marine Corps Community Services (MCCS) morale, welfare, and recreation programs. These can include individuals who work at fitness (gym), shopping (military exchanges), and recreation (golf courses, campgrounds, pools) facilities, as well as other service positions (e.g., car washes, gas stations, video stores). The program teaches these individuals to recognize and report individuals in distress. During the second day of training, participants design a sustainment plan to describe what they are going to do to keep using the active listening techniques they developed during the training. Most of the information for the training is excerpted from the Marine Corps Leaders Guide for Managing Marines in Distress (Werbel, 2009).

Programs for Caregivers. The Assessing and Managing Suicide Risk program was an optional one-day workshop for behavioral health-care providers and chaplains that taught strategies on how to assess and manage suicide risk. The training was developed collaboratively by the AAS and the SPRC. Training is delivered through lecture, video demonstrations, and exercises. A manual is also handed out to participants (Suicide Prevention Resource Center Training Institute, undated). In the Marine Corps, the current SPPM is the only person certified to deliver this training and conducts it on an ad hoc basis; however, in November 2009, there were no plans to sustain the training when the current SPPM leaves his post.

Programs for Deployed Personnel. The Operational Stress Control and Readiness (OSCAR) program began in 1999 and embeds behavioral health professionals into infantry regiments. Behavioral health professionals act as COSC specialists who educate and are educated by their marines through repeated contact in the field and shared experiences before, during, and after deployment (Nash, 2006). In November 2009, the program was not fully implemented, due to shortages in behavioral health professionals, and behavioral health professionals were being embedded in OSCAR teams on an ad hoc basis.

Postvention. The Marine Corps Personal Services Manual describes postvention services as "services targeted towards surviving family members, co-workers, and units after a suicide death of a service member" (MCO P1700.24B). Part of the command-level suicide-prevention program requires commands to provide support to the families after a suicide or suspected suicide. There are no standardized guidelines for commands on how to provide support or what types of support to provide. Upon request, Critical Incident Stress Debriefing (CISD) teams, which include chaplains and behavioral health professionals, are also available to assist units affected by the suicide of a member, through debriefings and social support. Finally, unit chaplains also provide support to families and units and provide counseling and assistance with memorial services (MCO P1700.24B).

Conclusion

As described, DoD and each service have a myriad of activities currently in place to prevent suicides. Consistent across the services is a strong reliance on universal prevention programs. Gatekeeper training specifically designed for leaders and chaplains is also common, but so too are programs that treat all servicemembers as potential gatekeepers. Means restriction is referenced only as a component of the Marine Corps suicide-prevention program (see Chapter Five), though there is little policy guidance on this topic. Also, while each service has in place organizations responsible for providing assistance after a servicemember takes his or her life, no formal postvention policies exist.

Support for Suicide Prevention in the Department of Defense

In this chapter, we provide detailed information on how suicide-prevention programming in DoD and for each service is supported. For each service, we provide information using the following organization:

1. *official documentation bearing on suicide:* We present the service-specific policies and instructions that bear directly on suicide or suicide prevention.
2. *organizations responsible for suicide prevention:* We describe the organizations and personnel deemed responsible, by policy or instruction for each specific service, for suicide prevention. For each service, this is described in three domains: headquarter level, installation level, and, when appropriate, organizations and personnel deemed responsible in theater.
3. *funding for suicide prevention:* We describe how suicide-prevention activities are funded.

Our service-specific descriptions across these domains derive from the review of materials and policy and expert interviews we conducted. When possible, we attempt to provide the same level of detail for each service. However, this is not always possible, as the level of information available across the services describing aspects of suicide-prevention activities varies. We provide an overview of this information graphically in Table 5.1, followed by descriptions for each service.

Support for Suicide Prevention in the Army

Official Documentation Bearing on Suicide in the Army

The Army Posture Statement (APS) includes information papers that describe specific initiatives that the Army is supporting to meet its overall goals and the reasoning behind its efforts. The APS thus includes information on the ASPP. The Suicide Prevention Information Paper, available on the Army's website, provides overarching goals for the ASPP:

Table 5.1
Support for Suicide Prevention, by Service

Type of Support	Army	Navy	Air Force	Marines
Policy	AR 600-63 DA PAM 600-24 AR 600-85 TRADOC PAM 600-22	OPNAVINST 1720.4A NAVADMINs	AFPAM 44-160 AFI 44-154 AFI 44-109 AFI 44-153 AFI 90-501 Health Services Inspection Guide[a] AF Guide for Managing Suicidal Behavior[b] Leader's Guide for Managing Personnel in Distress	MCO P1700.24B MCO P1700.27A MCO P1700.29 MCO P3040.4E MCRP 6-11C MCO 1510.89B MARADMINs
Organizations	Headquarters G-1[c] G-3 Surgeon General (CHPPM) Interim ASPTF Installations CHPC ISRT/SRT Gatekeepers (AR 600-63) MEDCOM Theater HSS CSC teams	Headquarters Education and Training Command Deputy Chief of Naval Operations[c] BUMED NMCPHC Installations Installation commanders SPC NOSC	Headquarters AF Suicide Prevention IPT Chief of Staff CAIB Surgeon General[c] Installations IDS TSR	Headquarters Personal and Family Readiness[c] Combat Development Command TRADOC Installations Installation commanders SPC
Funding	Recently dedicated funding (FY 2011) Internal organizational funds	Internal organizational funds Grants Dedicated funding	Internal organizational funds Dedicated funding	Dedicated funding

[a] U.S. Department of the Air Force (2006a).

[b] AFMOA (undated).

[c] SPPM is located here.

NOTE: AR = Army regulation. DA = Department of the Army. PAM = pamphlet. OPNAVINST = Office of the Chief of Naval Operations instruction. NAVADMIN = Navy administrative memorandum. AFPAM = Air Force pamphlet. MCO = Marine Corps order. MCRP = Marine Corps reference publication. MARADMIN = Marine Corps administrative memorandum. CHPC = Community Health Promotion Council. MEDCOM = U.S. Army Medical Command. HSS = Health Service Support. CSC = combat stress control. BUMED = Bureau of Medicine and Surgery. FY = fiscal year.

- Reduce the stigma of seeking mental health care.
- Improve access to behavioral health providers.
- Raise the awareness of junior leaders while instilling intervention skills.
- Provide actionable intelligence to field commanders that includes lessons learned and trend analysis.

- Increase life skills (U.S. Department of the Army, 2008a).[1]

Additionally, the APS information paper charts the path of the ASPP, from inception in 1984 through the recent increases in focus and push for a multidisciplinary approach to suicide prevention. While not a formal policy, the document summarizes important overarching goals for the ASPP. These overarching goals are contained in three Army regulations, described below.

AR 600-63, Army Health Promotion, was recently revised and includes information on the ASPP goals and objectives. Section 4-4 of this regulation establishes the policy and regulations for the ASPP, whose purpose is to minimize suicidal behavior and to establish a community approach to reduce Army suicides. This section stipulates that prevention programs will be implemented throughout the Army to secure the safety of individuals at risk for suicide, minimize the adverse effects of suicidal behavior on unit cohesion and other military personnel, and preserve mission effectiveness and warfighting capability. These goals are accomplished through five overarching prevention strategies that are similar to the "goals" within the APS:

- Develop positive life coping skills.
- Encourage help-seeking behavior.
- Raise awareness of and vigilance toward suicide prevention.
- Synchronize, integrate, and manage the ASPP.
- Conduct suicide surveillance, analysis, and reporting.

DA PAM 600-24, Health Promotion, Risk Reduction, and Suicide Prevention (December 17, 2009), complements AR 600-63 and provides holistic guidance to improving the physical, mental, and spiritual health of soldiers and their families. The pamphlet provides procedures for establishing the elements in its new title and was recently updated to include a description of suicide-prevention activities and efforts that emanated from the ASPTF. The previous version of the pamphlet was drawn from older versions of 600-63 and was revised recently within the Army.[2]

AR 600-85, The Army Substance Abuse Program, also addresses suicide directly.[3] The regulation makes reducing suicide a risk-reduction priority, along with other high-risk behaviors, such as substance abuse, spouse and child abuse, sexually transmitted

---

[1] The 2008 APS formed the basis of many changes to suicide prevention in the Army. Since then, much has happened. By 2010, the information paper on suicide prevention was changed to *Army Campaign Plan for Health Promotion, Risk Reduction and Suicide Prevention* (U.S. Department of the Army, 2010).

[2] Recent changes recommended by the ASPTF include updating roles and responsibilities of current organizations, including new organizations and task forces for administering suicide-prevention programs, standardizing nomenclature and training programs, and new policies and procedures for providing support to families.

[3] There is also a recent Expeditionary Substance Abuse Program (ESAP) in pilot testing, which aims to provide prevention and treatment services to deployed soldiers.

diseases, and crimes against property. The regulation, through the Army G-1, creates a Department of the Army Risk Reduction Program Working Group and codifies the command-level Risk Reduction Program (RRP) for implementation in installations with more than 500 active-duty soldiers. The objectives of the RRP are to compile, analyze, and assess behavioral risk and other data to identify trends and units with high-risk profiles. It also provides systematic prevention and intervention methods and materials to commanders to eliminate or mitigate individual high-risk behaviors.

TRADOC PAM 600-22, Leaders Guide for Suicide Prevention Planning, is an overarching pamphlet from TRADOC that provides a lay discussion of background material on suicides in the Army, short descriptions of leadership and community responsibilities, stigma associated with revealing suicidal thoughts and behaviors, and references containing additional information. The discussion in this pamphlet is similar in tone and content to a shorter, older, illustrated guide, *Guide to the Prevention of Suicide and Self-Destructive Behavior* (DA PAM 600-70).

Organizations Responsible for Suicide Prevention in the Army

Headquarters. Army G-1 serves as the Army staff proponent for the Army Health Promotion Program and has overarching responsibility for suicide prevention and particularly the ASPP, which is within DAPE-HRI (Human Resources). The SPPM is currently a GS-15. The Army's suicide-prevention programs are not all run through the ASPP, but rather span multiple organizations, which thus diffuses control for suicide-prevention activities and makes the ASPP a player in, though not necessarily the focal point for, all efforts.

Army G-3 contains a recently organized branch DAMO-CSF, which controls the Army's CSF program, which will include some suicide-prevention activities in the future.[4]

The Surgeon General's office addresses suicide prevention through various organizations, including CHPPM. CHPPM's Directorate of Health Promotion and Wellness maintains a website (CHPPM, 2010) with information and resources for suicide prevention. Products available from CHPPM are requested by or available to the ASPP, which can adopt and further promulgate them within the Army. CHPPM provides suicide-prevention materials as a service to the Army from internal funding of programs. An example is the Army's ACE program, which was created at CHPPM at the request of the G-1 and has been adopted within the Army to be a major component of suicide-prevention training.

In March 2009, the Army stood up the ASPTF, an interim organization charged with making urgent and lasting changes in the way the Army approaches health promotion, risk reduction, and suicide prevention. This task force, which was led by the Vice Chief of Staff of the Army and included representation from across the Army

---

[4]   See the CSF website (U.S. Army, undated).

staff, including personnel from the ASPP, was designed to provide immediate, coordinated reporting and programmatic solutions to reduce suicides within Army ranks. The task force analyzed existing health-promotion systems and processes within the Army to provide recommendations to take immediate actions to improve health, reduce risk, and prevent suicides. Specifically, the objectives of the task force were to reduce suicides within the Army and to produce an Army campaign plan for health promotion, risk reduction, and suicide prevention. The campaign plan was released in April 2009 (see Dahms, 2009) and included a list of tasks for agencies across the Army, including changing and updating current doctrine describing suicide prevention and related risk factors, assessing and analyzing current programs and organizations involved with suicide prevention, and developing metrics and other activities across the domains of doctrine, organization, training, materiel, leadership, personnel, and facilities (DOTMLPF).

Installations. Each garrison commander appoints a CHPC whose responsibility is to implement the health-promotion program and synchronize, integrate, and manage the installation suicide-prevention program (AR 600-63). The council is expected to meet at least quarterly. Among its duties is performing the following functions in support of suicide prevention:

- Ensure that suicide-prevention activities are carried out in accordance with Army regulations.
- Ensure that suicide-prevention programs are well advertised and promoted to leaders, organizations, and tenant units.
- Monitor the use of helping agencies (both external and internal to the installation) to identify trends.
- Coordinate with local community services in support of suicide prevention.
- Ensure that all gatekeepers are properly trained to recognize behavioral patterns that place individuals at risk for suicide.
- Identify installation-wide events that might increase the risk of suicide, and take appropriate measures.

Organizationally, the CHPC provides overarching guidance on suicide-prevention activities at the installation and establishes ISRTs/SRTs[5] to respond to any known or suspected suicide in tenant units through the ISRTs'/SRTs' support to unit commanders, ensure that guidelines are followed for local media coverage, and monitor completion and submission of the ASER (now referred to as DoDSER; see Chapter Four).

Unit commanders, chaplains, and behavioral health-care providers are responsible for implementing suicide-prevention awareness and training. Army regulations and

---

[5] ISRTs have recently been changed to SRTs, as of the most recent version of AR 600-63 (dated September 20, 2009).

training and awareness materials available on the G-1 website[6] identify whom soldiers should contact for additional information on suicide or to seek help.

Installation "gatekeepers" are assigned by the Army to essentially be the first line of defense in suicide intervention and prevention and provide specific counseling to soldiers and civilians in need (AR 600-63). Gatekeepers are further subdivided into primary and secondary grades. Primary gatekeepers are those people "whose primary duties involve assisting those in need who are more susceptible to suicide ideation," and secondary gatekeepers are those "who may have a secondary opportunity to come in contact with a person at risk" (AR 600-63). The gatekeepers are seen as first responders and typically receive additional training and accreditation to identify and address mental health problems that might lead to suicide. Table 5.2 lists some examples of the primary and secondary gatekeepers identified by the Army. Notably missing from the example gatekeeper list documented in AR 600-63 are a soldier's peers, who have been the focus of the recent ACE training. In garrison, the Army specifies gatekeepers who include family life chaplains, Army Community Service, medical services, marriage and family counselors, and postdeployment centers. During combat, combat stress control teams are used as the points of contact, along with medics, Battalion Aid Stations, and chaplains.

The gatekeepers on post are trained for different levels of suicide-prevention activities. AR 600-63 identifies suicide-prevention training to be conducted by and for specific organizations. For example, as an identified gatekeeper, chaplains and their assistants in Unit Ministry Teams assist commanders to provide suicide-prevention and awareness training for soldiers, Army civilians, and family members in their respective units and communities. All chaplains and assistants receive basic and advanced suicide-prevention and awareness training as determined by the Chief of Chaplains. As of 2002, this training included ASIST workshops and interactive electronic materials to reinforce training. The chaplains are also to consult with local behavioral health-

Table 5.2
Examples of Primary and Secondary Gatekeepers

Primary Gatekeepers	Secondary Gatekeepers
Chaplains and chaplain assistants	Military police
ASAP counselors	Trial defense lawyers
Family Advocacy Program workers	Inspectors general
Army Emergency Relief counselors	DoD school counselors
Emergency-room medical technicians	Red Cross workers
Medical and dental health professionals	First-line supervisors

SOURCE: AR 600-63.
NOTE: ASAP = Army Substance Abuse Program.

---

[6]   See, for example, "Suicide Awareness for Leaders 2007" (Deputy Chief of Staff, 2009b).

care providers to ensure that information provided to units is scientifically and medically accurate.

Behavioral health professionals provide health promotion, prevention, and clinical services to address suicidal and self-injurious behaviors. MEDCOM is tasked to ensure that uniformed behavioral health-care providers receive initial training as part of residency and fellowship programs sponsored by MEDCOM or as part of the advanced training portion of the Basic Officer Leadership Course. Refresher and update training is available to uniformed behavioral health-care professionals through the Behavioral Science Short Course; however, attendance is not currently required.

Theater. The HSS system provides in-theater support for suicide prevention. The HSS is broadly divided into five levels of care, from level 1 emergency treatment performed by brigade and below units on the battlefield through health providers assigned to the units (e.g., organic), to level 5 care at medical treatment facilities in the United States (see Table 5.3 for a breakdown of those levels) (FM 4-0; JP 1-02). The main provider of behavioral health services on the battlefield is included in the mental health sections of medical companies, organic elements at the division level, separate brigade personnel, and the area support medical battalion; all these units change in numbers and types of personnel, depending on the mission.

CSC teams provide additional support to medical companies. The Army's CSC efforts involve behavioral health personnel who are a part of brigade and above units. CSC teams are available from CSC detachments or companies to provide specific augmentation as needed (FM 22-51). The teams have their own vehicles to move forward to augment the tactical units or to support combat service support units over a wide area. Each CSC detachment supports one division or two to three separate brigades

Table 5.3
Five Levels of the Health Service Support System for the Army

Level	Description
1	Treatment by trauma/emergency care specialists Immediate lifesaving measures Disease and nonbattle-injury prevention
2 (division level)	Operated by treatment platoon of medical companies and troops Advanced trauma and EMT capabilities Patients with RTD of <3 days are treated Preventive medicine and COSC assets are colocated
3	MTF staffed and equipped for all patients
4	MTF that may not be in theater of operations
5	CONUS-based medical care

SOURCE: Adapted from FM 4-0.

NOTE: EMT = emergency medical technician. RTD = return to duty. CONUS = continental United States.

or regiments (AMEDD, 2008). It consists of three four-person CSC preventive teams that move forward to brigade support areas when requested and one 11-person combat stress fitness (restoration) team that can run a "combat fitness center" in the division support area or the corps forward area. The team also provides preventive services to units in their vicinity and can go further forward.

Each CSC company (see Figure 5.1) includes six CSC prevention (CSCP) teams and four combat stress fitness (restoration) (CSCR) teams. It supports the corps units behind two or three divisions but can send teams far forward to augment the division rear and even brigades in combat, similar to what the CSC detachments do.

Funding for Suicide Prevention in the Army

Suicide prevention in the Army has historically been funded through internal organizational funds within the G-1 and elsewhere. For instance, there was no programmatic funding for the ASPP within G-1. Materials produced within CHPPM are typically generated from internal funds within specific directorates. According to the Suicide Prevention Program Office within the G-1, there are plans to move toward a more centralized funding mechanism for suicide prevention in coming years. As of this writing, some suicide-prevention activities have been added as a budget item in the FY 2011 budget.

Figure 5.1
Organizational Structure of a Combat Stress Control Company

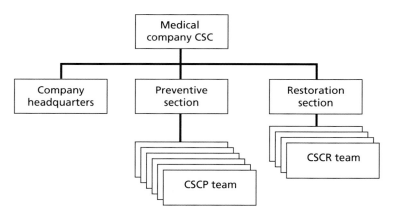

NOTE: CSCP = CSC prevention. CSCR = CSC restoration.
RAND MG953-5.1

Support for Suicide Prevention in the Navy

Official Documentation Bearing on Suicide in the Navy

OPNAVINST 1720.4A was issued in 2009 and established the U.S. Navy suicide-prevention program as part of official policy.[7] These instructions outlined the Navy's action plan to prevent suicides, which is comprised of eight elements:

- Command will conduct annual suicide-prevention training for all sailors that instructs individuals how to self-identify and identify peers at risk for suicide.
- Commanding officers (COs) will appoint an SPC to advise commands on suicide-prevention and crisis response programs.
- Senior leadership will publish messages stating that it is concerned about the risk of suicide among sailors.
- Command-level suicide-prevention and crisis response programs and associated action plans will be developed to provide education and increase awareness and referral of at-risk individuals.
- Chaplains and medical and behavioral health personnel shall provide unit-level expertise and coordinate plans and programs.
- Suicide prevention will be included in Life Skills training.
- The Navy will provide support to families and units adversely affected by suicide.
- The Navy will collect data and conduct an epidemiological analysis post–suicide event.

NAVADMINs, administrative messages sent out by email to all naval personnel to address pressing issues as needed, were used to issue relevant messages. Three of these deal specifically with procedural issues related to suicide prevention:

- NAVADMIN 243/05 was issued in September 2005 in support of the Navy suicide-prevention programs. The statement indicated that suicide was not a taboo subject and must be openly discussed. It aimed to debunk misconceptions that people who threaten suicide do not go on to kill themselves and that suicides happen only during the holidays. It advertised the support network (emergency care centers, mental health clinics, substance-abuse rehabilitation programs, FFSCs, military chaplains or civilian clergy) and the suicide-prevention video "Suicide Awareness: Making the Critical Decision" (MCCS, undated [b]). This message also reinforced the requirement that all COs provide training on suicide prevention at least annually and have a local plan for managing individuals who "present suicidal ideations, intents, or plans" (NAVADMIN 243/05).

---

[7]   OPNAVINST 1720.4A was updated on August 4, 2009.

- NAVADMIN 033/09 was released in January 2009 and required all naval personnel to complete the training course "Introduction to the Stress Continuum and Suicide Awareness" (NAVADMIN 033/09).
- NAVADMIN 122/09, issued in April 2009, directed the collection of data on Navy suicides for all active and reserve components and defines *suicide* as a self-inflicted death with evidence, either implicit or explicit, of intent to die; a *suicide attempt* as a self-inflicted, potentially injurious behavior with a nonfatal outcome for which there is evidence of intent to die; and other suicidal behaviors (i.e., expressed suicide-related thoughts, communications, and nonfatal self-injurious behavior without evidence of intent to die). NAVADMIN 122/09 also requires that all naval MTFs and the naval force command and RC commands appoint a DoDSER POC responsible for reporting data on suicides, suicide attempts, and other suicide behaviors (NAVADMIN 122/09).

Organizations Responsible for Suicide Prevention in the Navy

Headquarters. The Commander of NETC is responsible for providing a curriculum for annual suicide-prevention training and ensuring that suicide-prevention training tailored to sailors at each level of leadership is delivered through leadership courses of instruction (e.g., Officer Candidate School, Officer Development School). The commander is also responsible for including suicide intervention training in the curriculum used to train hospital corpsmen, religious specialists, and military police.

The Deputy Chief of Naval Operations for Manpower, Personnel, Training and Education is responsible for establishing a suicide-prevention program policy. Also within the Office of the Chief of Naval Operations, Personal Readiness and Community Support is responsible for developing policy guidance for suicide prevention; providing educational support (e.g., training materials, posters), and training to commands and SPCs; and monitoring the number of suicides by coordinating a database with the Navy casualty office, the OAFME, the DCoE, and the BUMED director of Psychological Health for Navy Reserve. The database should provide statistical data to inform ongoing program evaluation and the chain of command.

The Navy's SPPM is located within the Personal Readiness and Community Support branch. The position is a secondary duty that is done in addition to the prevention manager's primary duties and is currently held by a psychologist whose primary duty is program manager of the Navy's Behavioral Health Program.

The Chief of Chaplains, part of the Navy Annex, is responsible for developing policies and procedures that ensure that chaplains help commands implement and evaluate the suicide-prevention program (as requested) and consults with BUMED on policies related to chaplains' screening and assessment of sailors' suicidal behavior. Commands can also request assistance from the Chief of Chaplains with implementing and evaluating their suicide-prevention programming.

A captain under the Chief of Naval Personnel currently serves as program coordinator to the OSC program (described in detail in Chapter Four).

BUMED is the headquarters for Navy Medicine, and the Surgeon General of the Navy serves as the Chief of BUMED. He or she is responsible for policies and procedures that ensure that medical personnel use proper screening, assessment, and treatment techniques with sailors exhibiting suicidal behaviors and that DoDSERs are completed for suicide attempts.[8] The Chief of BUMED is also responsible for ensuring that MTFs have written protocols on suicide prevention maintained in acute-care areas and emergency rooms. Staff from BUMED's Deployment Health Support Directorate also assist in running the OSC program and are developing official doctrine to support this program.

The NMCPHC is located within the Navy Medicine Support Command, one of the four regional commands that support Navy Medicine. The NMCPHC assists in developing and disseminating messages on suicide awareness to all sailors through newsletters, posters, brochures, and videos.

Installations. The Commander, Navy Installations Command, is responsible for ensuring that emergency response personnel receive annual training on safety precautions and deescalation techniques when responding to sailors exhibiting potential suicide-related behaviors. COs are responsible for establishing and maintaining a suicide-prevention program that includes a designated SPC.

SPCs at each installation receive training from Personal Readiness and Community Support and are responsible for advising the chain of command on issues related to suicide prevention, as well as scheduling and conducting suicide-prevention training. Although not every installation has yet appointed an SPC, those that do have them often appoint chaplains or counselors from FFSCs.

Within each unit, chaplains are also available to counsel sailors in distress. On installations, sailors can access behavioral health providers and programs (e.g., substance-abuse rehabilitation program, the safe harbor program for individuals severely or very severely ill or injured) and FFSCs and naval health clinics, hospitals, and medical centers.[9] In addition, several interviewees mentioned that the OSC program is line owned and led, meaning that responsibility for OSC training is infused throughout the operational chain of command from top-level leadership to the front-line leaders, and is supported by chaplains, FFSCs, and front-line leaders (petty officers and junior officers) within each unit.

Within each Navy OSC (i.e., centers located in each state, each of which houses a command ombudsman who serves as the POC for reservists), Psychological Health

---

[8]   According to OPNAVINST 1720.4A, the Deputy Chief of Naval Operations is responsible for monitoring the number of suicides and tracking trends of all completed suicides in the Navy.

[9]   Many of these same or comparable resources are available within Army, Air Force, and Marine Corps units; the Navy officially recognizes these as responsible for suicide prevention in OPNAVINST 1720.4A.

Outreach Coordinators, via the Psychological Health Outreach Program, provide assessment and referral and coordinate care and follow-up for reservists receiving services from MTFs, clinics and hospitals run by the VHA, and civilian providers. The Psychological Health Outreach Program also offers health education (e.g., training on OSC, workshops for returning sailors to address deployment stress) to all reservists.

Funding for Suicide Prevention in the Navy

Each of the organizations that conduct suicide-prevention initiatives independently funds these activities. Two of the initiatives (i.e., the Reserve Psychological Health Outreach program and the RWW) are grant funded through supplemental funding released to the Navy by the U.S. Troop Readiness, Veterans' Care, Katrina Recovery, and Iraq Accountability Appropriations Act of 2007 (Pub. L. 110-28). Aside from these grants, there is limited dedicated funding. Although suicide prevention is not a line item in the budget, there is a modest amount of dedicated funding for behavioral health. We were told that suicide prevention in the Navy competes for resources and staff time with other initiatives, including tobacco-use prevention, stress management, and psychological health, and that "no assigned budget means we have to fight for resources."

We were informed that the FY 2010 Navy budget would contain a line item of $82,000 in funding dedicated to suicide prevention. This funding will cover printing of posters and brochures and travel for the Navy SPPM and another staff member to conduct training on suicide prevention at the professional development conferences for first responders, installation SPCs, and chaplains. In FY 2010, BUMED will also fund two supplemental suicide-prevention initiatives: the Assessing and Managing Suicide Risk workshop for mental health professionals, counselors, and chaplains, and travel for all installation SPCs to attend a two-day training conference.

Support for Suicide Prevention in the Air Force

Official Documentation Bearing on Suicide in the Air Force

AFPAM 44-160, The Air Force Suicide Prevention Program, describes in detail the 11 initiatives of the AFSPP.

AFI 44-154, Suicide and Violence Prevention Education and Training, describes the requirements for suicide-prevention training.

Section LD 3.4.3 of the Health Services Inspection Guide, 2006, IDS/CAIB/ Suicide Prevention, establishes inspection criteria for Air Force Medical Service (AFMS) related to suicide-prevention policy (U.S. Department of the Air Force, 2006a).

AFI 44-109, Mental Health, Confidentiality and Military Law, establishes rules for confidentiality, defines conditions requiring communication between mental health providers and commanders, and expands the scope of the LPSP program.

AFI 44-153, Traumatic Stress Response (TSR), outlines the requirements for TSR (formerly known as Critical Incident Stress Management), one of the 11 initiatives of AFSPP.

AFI 90-501, Community Action Information Board and Integrated Delivery System, outlines responsibilities and requirements of the CAIBs and the IDS.

Air Force Guide for Managing Suicidal Behavior: Strategies, Resources, and Tools (AFMOA, undated) is a guide for clinicians on managing suicidal behavior. This guide was published in 2004 and stems from the Managing Behavior Project initiated in the Air Force in 2002. Also related to the Managing Behavior Project, in 2007, the Air Force contracted with the SPRC to train behavioral health staff (psychologists, psychiatrists, and social workers) in the Air Force on managing suicidal behavior in clinical practice (AFMOA, undated).

In addition, memoranda from the Chief of Staff, Vice Chief of Staff, and Surgeon General are regularly sent to all MAJCOMs and AFMS staff in order to inform them of changes in suicide-prevention policy and remind them of the importance of suicide prevention. These memoranda are available on the AFSPP website (U.S. Air Force, undated).

Organizations Responsible for Suicide Prevention in the Air Force

Headquarters. The Air Force Suicide Prevention IPT created the suicide-prevention program in the U.S. Air Force (USAF). As specifically described in AFPAM 44-160, the IPT consisted of representatives of military and civilian personnel, chaplains, Safety, Staff Judge Advocate, commanders, first sergeants, Child and Youth Programs, Family Support, Family Advocacy, law enforcement, Office of Special Investigations, epidemiology, mental health, and preventive medicine, as well as individuals from the CDC, the Armed Forces Institute of Pathology, and the Walter Reed Army Institute of Research (AFPAM 44-160). The formal IPT no longer meets; however, the CAIB or AF/CC charters a working group when an issue of need for a specific program arises.

The AF/CC disseminates information about the suicide-prevention program to Air Force commanders and personnel in order to establish its importance and ensure that information is received in a timely manner and by leadership at all levels (AFPAM 44-160).

CAIBs were established to provide a formal management structure and oversight for the AFSPP outside of the Suicide Prevention IPT (AFI 90-501). A CAIB exists at the headquarters, MAJCOM, and installation levels. The CAIB at Air Force Headquarters is chaired by the Assistant Vice Chief of Staff. Membership includes representatives from the Deputy Chief of Staff for Manpower and Personnel (AF/A1) (Airman and Family Readiness Centers, formerly termed Community Support and Family Readiness); Air Force Chaplain Corps (AF/HC) (Plans and Programs Division); Air Force Deputy Chief of Staff for Logistics, Installations and Mission Support

(AF/A4/7) (Family Member Program); Air Force Judge Advocate (AF/JA); Air Force Reserve (AF/RE); Air Force Safety (AF/SE); Air Force Surgeon General (AF/SG); Deputy Chief of Staff, Air, Space and Information Operations, Plans and Requirements (AF/A3/5); Director of the Air National Guard (NGB/CF); Air Force Command Chief Master Sergeant (AF/CCC); Secretary of the Air Force for Budget (SAF/FMB); Secretary of the Air Force for Force Management Integration (SAF/MRM); and Secretary of the Air Force for Public Affairs (SAF/PA).

The AF/SG disseminates information pertaining to clinical aspects of the suicide-prevention program to AFMS staff and Air Force personnel. The Surgeon General is also a member of the CAIB.

The Air Force SPPM resides within the office of the Surgeon General. The SPPM is assigned full time to suicide prevention, though he or she may occasionally have collateral responsibility for other programs. He or she is responsible for compiling up-to-date suicide statistics among airmen and manages the AFSPP, and represents the Air Force on the SPARRC.

Installations. Commanders are responsible for passing information on suicide prevention from the AF/CC to their subordinates.

Installation CAIBs are chaired by the installation commander and are comprised of a support group commander, medical group commander, operations group commander, maintenance group commander, staff judge advocate, senior chaplain, civil engineering commander, public affairs officer, services squadron commander, comptroller squadron commander, security forces squadron commander, mission support squadron commander, Air Reserve Component commanders, and CCC (AFI 90-501). These organizations serve as a forum for cross-organizational review and resolution of individual, family, and installation community issues.

The IDS is a standing subcommittee of the CAIB that develops a comprehensive and coordinated plan for integrating community outreach and prevention programs, including suicide prevention (AFI 90-501). The Air Force IDS consists of representatives from all AF functional communities represented on the AF CAIB.

TSR (formerly Critical Incident Stress Management) exists at every installation and consists of behavioral health-care providers, medical providers, chaplains, and senior NCOs in nonmedical positions (AFI 44-153). Their primary role is to assist personnel in confronting their reactions to traumatic incidents, including suicide.

Funding for Suicide Prevention in the Air Force

For the past two fiscal years, approximately $200,000 has been specifically budgeted annually for suicide prevention. In addition, training products may be funded by access to additional psychological health money. CAIB and IDS activities are cross-functional forums and do not have assigned budgets; thus, funding is provided by participating agencies and supplemented by CAIB chair resources when necessary.

Support for Suicide Prevention in the Marine Corps

The U.S. Marine Corps is part of the Department of the Navy; the Commandant of the Marine Corps, the most senior officer in the Marine Corps, reports directly to the Secretary of the Navy. Navy medical and dental personnel, as well as chaplains, support Marines. It is important to keep this organizational structure in mind when reviewing this section, as the Marine Corps and the Navy share resources and regulations related to suicide prevention.

Official Documentation Bearing on Suicide in the Marine Corps

MCO P1700.24B, the Marine Corps Personal Services Manual, established the Marine Corps suicide-prevention program as a policy in 2001. The Personal Services Manual outlines policies that guide mobility support programs (e.g., successful relocations, transition to civilian life), counseling services (e.g., marriage and family counseling), and prevention programs, including suicide prevention. This policy lists suicide prevention as a required program, and the program is defined in the Personal Services Manual as consisting of eight components:

- *Awareness Education and Health Promotion:* Commanders communicate to all marines about suicide prevention and ensure that all marines receive annual suicide awareness and prevention training and health promotion through the Semper Fit fitness program.
- *Life Skills Training:* The purpose of Life Skills Training is to reduce the incidence of problems that detract from personal and unit readiness, such as alcohol abuse and stress.
- *Leadership Training:* This provides leaders at all levels with information and skills to improve their identification of and intervention with at-risk personnel.
- *Crisis Intervention and Risk Management:* This establishes procedures that detail how to refer and evaluate a marine with behavioral health problems, how to provide crisis care (e.g., suicide watches), and procedures for restricting access to lethal means.[10]
- *Counseling and Treatment:* This provides services and programs to address personal, family, and mental health issues that contribute to suicidal behavior.
- *Postvention Services:* These provide support to families and units affected by suicide.
- *Casualty Reporting and Trend Analysis:* This provides incident reports to inform research on the risk and protective factors related to suicide. Incident reports are also reviewed to improve future prevention efforts.

---

[10] Although the Personal Services Manual lists restricting access to lethal means as a component of the suicide-prevention program, we found no specialized policy or procedure to support any restrictions.

- *Inspections:* This requires regularly inspecting commanding generals' completion and recording of the annual suicide awareness and prevention training.

MCO P1700.27A, the Marine Corps Community Services Policy Manual, requires that health-promotion officers integrate health-promotion elements into the Semper Fit program, including positive lifestyle and behavior changes.

MCO P1700.29, the Marine Corps Semper Fit Program Manual, includes suicide awareness as one of its nine educational elements.

MCO P3040.4E, the Marine Corps Casualty Procedures Manual, designates that suicide attempts or gestures or suicides of active-duty marines should be reported, as should deaths of reserve marines who die under nonhostile conditions.

MCRP 6-11C, the Marine Corps Combat Stress manual, includes suicide awareness materials, such as how to recognize signs of suicide and steps for prevention.

MCO 1510.89B, volume 1 of the Individual Training Standard (ITS) System for Marine Corps Common Skills, is "written for all Military Occupational Specialties (MOS) in order to specify the critical skills required by units of their individual Marines in support of the unit." Explaining steps necessary in the prevention of suicide is now listed as an ITS, though it is not clear what MOSs are required to obtain this ITS.

MARADMINs—administrative messages that go to the entire Marine Corps and augment policy—have gone out to address suicide-related issues in 2008–2009. Following is a brief summary of the directive MARADMINs that describe a change in procedures related to suicide:

- MARADMIN 147/08 required that the DoDSER be completed for all suicides beginning January 1, 2008.
- MARADMIN 364/09 provided a summary of results from the 20th Executive Safety Board (ESB) meeting. The ESB, chaired by the Assistant Commandant of Marine Corps and comprised of 20 two- or three-star generals, meets every six months to discuss pressing safety concerns. Suicide awareness and prevention were covered during the October 2008 ESB, and the MARADMIN that described the ESB results detailed two suicide-prevention activities: (1) an NCO leadership training program to identify and assist marines at risk for suicide and (2) a leadership video with suicide prevention as part of its message.
- MARADMIN 404/09 and MARADMIN 436/09 provided implementation guidance for the NCO Suicide Prevention course. These messages contained procedures for how and when to conduct the train-the-trainer courses and follow-on training. Master training teams were instructed to train instructors (sergeants) at the battalion and unit levels. The MARADMINs also instructed trained sergeants to train all NCOs and Navy corpsmen immediately, with October 30,

2009, as a deadline for training all NCOs in the Marine Corps and all Navy corpsmen serving in Marine Corps units.

- MARADMIN 596/09 required all commands to designate a POC to receive and administer program evaluation materials for all NCO suicide-prevention courses.
- MARADMIN 134/09 required that every marine participate in a two-hour training for suicide prevention presented by leaders, the CO, and the executive officer of each unit. This MARADMIN communicated that, by March 15, 2009, every CO (colonel and above) had to produce a suicide-prevention video using local funds. To support this MARADMIN, TECOM provided an instruction guide for training, some sample slides, a description of messages that should be communicated in the video, and a sample video.[11] The message did not indicate how often this training should be administered.

Organizations Responsible for Suicide Prevention in the Marine Corps

Headquarters. The SPPM is a Behavioral Health Affairs Officer and is currently a Navy commander who is a clinical psychologist located within the Personal and Family Readiness Division of Marine Corps Headquarters (HQMC). The SPPM is dedicated full time to the suicide-prevention program and is responsible for overseeing the policy and program development related to suicide prevention for the entire Marine Corps. We were informed that there are currently five full-time staff members at HQMC working on suicide prevention: the SPPM, a master gunnery sergeant (E-9) specially assigned to manage the MCSPP, two program analysts, and an administrative support specialist, with no plans for additional hires.

COSC is a branch of the Personal and Family Readiness Division located in the Manpower and Reserve Affairs Department. It is staffed by a coordinator, deputy coordinator, and administrative staff person and supported by a multidisciplinary team of adjunct staff drawn from HQMC departments, Marine Corps Combat Development Command, operational commands, BUMED, the Navy chaplaincy, the VA, and the National Center for PTSD. Although not specific to suicide, COSC programs are delivered at each installation to prevent, identify, and holistically treat mental injuries caused by combat or other operations.

Marine Corps Combat Development Command is charged with research activities to inform HQMC suicide-prevention program development and is in the process of conducting a suicide-prevention literature review; developing recommendations for a data-collection approach to account for various USMC activities and agencies dealing with behavioral health, counseling, and support; and analyzing the effectiveness of existing programs.

TECOM is located under the *Deputy Commandant, Combat Development and Integration* (HQMC, undated). According to the Personal Services Manual, TECOM

---

[11] These materials are available from TECOM (undated).

is responsible for providing training on suicide risk factors and identifying and referring marines at risk for suicide to all officers, drill instructors, and permanent personnel (MCO P1700.24B). Periodic risk assessments and suicide awareness and prevention training during the recruit training cycle are also the responsibility of TECOM. Finally, TECOM must provide suicide awareness and prevention training to all officer candidates and all officers attending the Marine Corps University and ensure that suicide awareness and prevention training is incorporated into the curriculum of all formal leadership schools.

Installations. The Personal Services Manual requires that each installation command have a suicide-prevention program (MCO P1700.24B). As part of that program, commands are required to conduct annual suicide awareness training for all marines under their command, provide postvention support, and report on suicides. The Marine Corps encourages but does not specify what a command-level suicide-prevention program should contain. However, commanders are provided a copy of the Automated Inspection Reporting System (AIRS) checklist that outlines command requirements. Installation commanders are specifically responsible for the following (MCO P1700.24B):

- using local resources to establish an integrated program to educate all marines and identify, refer, treat, and follow up with at-risk marines. Local resources include leaders, medical staff, chaplains, Semper Fit coordinators, and Personal Services and Substance Abuse Counseling Center counselors.
- providing annual training in suicide awareness and prevention
- ensuring that leaders who provide annual training demonstrate current knowledge about suicide prevention, use standardized training materials, and offer up-to-date information about local resources
- following appropriate procedures for screening, evaluation, disposition, and treatment of all personnel deemed at risk for harm to themselves or others
- ensuring that all personnel at risk for harm to self or others are kept in sight and escorted to an evaluation with a competent medical authority and that all personnel who make suicide gestures or attempts are evaluated by a behavioral health professional and appropriate follow-up appointments are completed by referred personnel
- ensuring that a Personnel Casualty Report (PCR) is submitted on all suicides, attempts, and gestures
- coordinating with all military and civilian authorities to complete appropriate investigations or inquiries into all cases of suspected suicide by active-duty Marine Corps personnel

- completing a DoDSER on all cases of suicide deaths or undetermined deaths in which suicide has not been excluded[12]
- providing support to the families after a suicide or suspected suicide and using the CISD teams, as appropriate, to assist units affected by the suicide of a member
- encouraging leadership practices that promote prevention and the resolution of problems at the lowest possible level.

At each installation with at least 1,000 marines, there is a full-time staff position for an SPC as well as coordinators to serve reserve headquarters, recruiting command headquarters, and the Marine Corps combat development center. Installation-level SPCs serve as points of contact for HQMC staff to funnel relevant information and as resources to the commander of each installation. As of November 2009, we were told that hiring of installation suicide-prevention staff was still ongoing. There are additional suicide program officers (SPOs) who are members of specific units and who occupy the role as collateral duty. SPOs are responsible for implementing suicide-prevention activities at the unit level.

Funding for Suicide Prevention in the Marine Corps
Funding for suicide prevention comes from HQMC, which interviewees reported supports the previously described five full-time staff dedicated to suicide prevention and the suicide-prevention activities initiated through HQMC's Manpower and Reserve Affairs and TECOM. Manpower and Reserve Affairs provides training staff for the Are You Listening program (described in Chapter Four and Appendix D). The COSC and OSCAR initiatives, as well as the installation-level suicide-prevention program (including the assigned suicide-prevention program officers), are also supported by the Manpower and Reserve Affairs Personal and Family Readiness Division. Interviewees indicated that TECOM provided funds to the Martial Arts Center of Excellence in Quantico for staff to develop a suicide-prevention module for the Marine Corps Martial Arts Program (MCMAP) in consultation with the SPPM.

---

[12] Although completing the DONSIR is still listed as a command requirement on the AIRS, MARADMIN 147/08 required that the DoDSER be completed for all suicides beginning January 1, 2008.

CHAPTER SIX

Conclusions and Recommendations

The Six Essential Components of a Comprehensive Suicide-Prevention Program

Our review of the literature and interviews with experts in the field led us to conclude that a comprehensive suicide-prevention program has six essential components:

1. It raises awareness and promotes self-care.
2. It identifies those at high risk of suicide.
3. It facilitates access to quality care.
4. It provides quality care.
5. It restricts access to lethal means.
6. It responds appropriately to suicides and suicide attempts.

Our investigation into the suicide-prevention programs in DoD and across the services revealed examples of programs that fall under some of these domains. However, initiatives or activities were lacking in other domains. In this chapter, we describe our assessment of how DoD and the services are performing across each of these domains, represented graphically in Table 6.1.

Raise Awareness and Promote Self-Care

The services use three distinct strategies to raise awareness and promote self-care: media campaigns (including but not limited to websites, brochures, and posters), training and educational courses, and messages from key personnel, including leaders at both head-quarter and command levels. Most of the information conveyed through these dissemination vehicles raises awareness by publicizing suicide statistics, known risk factors for suicide, and resources for those considering suicide or in more-general distress, or by emphasizing the importance of suicide prevention. Such campaigns are noteworthy, as they are known to affect recipients' knowledge and attitudes about suicide and suicide prevention. The impact of awareness-raising campaigns on preventing actual suicides or promoting changes in behavior, however, is less evident.

Table 6.1
Assessment of Suicide-Prevention Activities Across Services

Goal	Army	Navy	Air Force	Marines
Raise awareness and promote self-care	Primarily awareness campaigns, with fewer initiatives aimed at promoting self-care			
Identify those at risk	Expansive but rely mostly on gatekeepers	Mostly rely on gatekeepers	Investigation policy	Mostly rely on gatekeepers
Facilitate access to quality care	Stigma addressed primarily by locating behavioral health care in nontraditional settings			
	No policy to assuage privacy or professional concerns		Limited privilege	No policy
	No education about benefits of accessing behavioral health care			
Deliver quality care	Not considered in domain of suicide prevention		Past efforts exist with a sustainment plan	Past efforts exist, but not sustained
Restrict access to lethal means	No current policies exist		Limited guidance	No policy
Respond appropriately	Personnel/teams available, but limited guidance			

Within the purview of suicide prevention, there are fewer messages disseminated with respect to promoting self-care. Most self-care messages across the services are conveyed in training or courses focused on building resiliency among those about to deploy or those returning from deployment. The Navy and Air Force also encourage members of those services to seek care early, before mild levels of distress escalate. Few programs actually teach strategies to help servicemembers build skills that would help them care for themselves, including the ability to self-refer when needed.

Identify Those at High Risk

All of the services have programs in place to identify those at elevated risk of suicide. The Army, Navy, and Marines have a variety of programs that train individuals to act as "gatekeepers," which entails recognizing the signs of peers or subordinates in distress, confronting the individual suspected to be at increased risk, and actively referring those in distress to follow-up care. The persons trained to serve as gatekeepers across these services range from other servicemembers to family members, commanders, and chaplains, and, in the Marine Corps, even front-desk clerks at fitness centers. While gatekeeper training may be intuitively appealing, there is insufficient evidence to date indicating that these training programs are effective at reducing suicides. Thus, more evaluation is needed.

An alternative strategy for identifying those at high risk of suicide is to monitor the aftermath of high-risk events. The Air Force actively includes this as a component of its suicide-prevention strategy by requiring that Air Force investigators notify an airman's commander, first sergeant, or supervisor through person-to-person contact that the airman was interviewed and notified that he or she was under investigation. Those appearing emotionally distraught after an interview will be released only to their commander, first sergeant, or supervisor.

Since deployment is associated with an increased risk of mental illness among servicemembers (Hoge, Castro, et al., 2004; Smith et al., 2008) and mental illness is one of the strongest risk factors for suicide, deployment can also be considered a high-risk event. The Army, Navy, and Air Force all have programs that attempt to monitor servicemembers after deployment and to mitigate the adverse consequences of deployment, though none of these programs has yet been associated with reductions in suicides or other suicidal behavior.

One of the more promising approaches for identifying those at high risk is through screening for mental health conditions in primary care. MEDCOM has directed widespread implementation of one such program, Re-Engineering Systems of Primary Care Treatment in the Military (RESPECT-Mil), in 15 Army MTFs (42 primary-care clinics). Other programs that promote mental health screening in primary care may exist across the services but were not considered under the umbrella of suicide-prevention activities by the key informants we interviewed.

Finally, some experts we interviewed thought that screening specifically for suicide risk by behavioral health-care providers was a promising practice. However, to date, such a practice has yet to be shown to reduce suicides, and the U.S. Preventive Task Force currently makes no recommendation with respect to screening for suicide risk. Nonetheless, the Air Force and Marine Corps have both offered one-time training programs for providers in suicide risk assessment and management, and the Air Force has developed an informal sustainment plan, including a published guide for behavioral health-care providers on managing suicidal behavior.

The identification of risk factors for suicide risk specifically within military populations can help guide the development of programs aimed at identifying those at high risk. A few research activities currently under way deserve mention, as they may provide useful information in this domain. The Army's Mental Health Advisory Teams (MHATs) have published six reports on the mental health conditions among soldiers in theater and, at the time of the writing of this monograph, were preparing a seventh investigation. In collaboration with NIMH, the Army has also recently initiated a research agenda focused on suicide.[1] The Air Force also has a program in which unit commanders can request an assessment of unit strengths and areas of vulnerabilities

---

[1]   The Marines are in discussions to join this initiative, though, as of January 6, 2010, no formal agreement between the organizations was yet in place.

across a range of behavioral factors that may increase the risk of suicide. All of these initiatives are well poised to provide valuable information on suicide risk.

Facilitate Access to Quality Care

Facilitating access to quality care involves overcoming the barriers that prevent military personnel from accessing behavioral health care. These barriers can generally be divided into three areas: stigma associated with accessing such care; concerns that accessing such care will harm their military careers or not be kept confidential; and beliefs that treatment is ineffective or that the prescription drugs used to treat mental health conditions have severe adverse side effects.

Across the services, most of the initiatives in place to facilitate access to quality care fall under the domain of eliminating stigma. For example, the initiatives that raise awareness about suicide and promote self-care are components of stigma reduction strategies. In addition, each service has programs in place in which behavioral health-care providers are located in nontraditional settings, including in primary care and in theater. Policy, such as the creation of the ASPTF, can also help convey the importance of suicide prevention and help reduce stigma associated with behavioral health care.

There are fewer initiatives focused on assuaging servicemembers' career and privacy concerns. Marine Corps leaders are instructed to convey to those in their charge that accessing behavioral health care will not harm them professionally. Air Force personnel are trained that voluntary mental health appointments are confidential in most cases and will not negatively harm their careers. The Air Force also has a limited-privilege program, whereby the information revealed to a behavioral health-care provider by those under investigation and deemed eligible for the program may not be used to characterize service at the time of an airman's separation. Aside from the Real Warriors campaign, which is a recently launched DoD-wide awareness campaign that includes videos of people describing the benefits they received from behavioral health care, there are few initiatives under the purview of suicide prevention in any of the services that seek to dispel myths about the ineffectiveness of behavioral health care.

Provide Quality Care to Those in Need

As described in detail in Chapter Three, the provision of quality care is a fundamental component of suicide prevention. It was beyond the scope of the current research project to evaluate the quality of care offered by behavioral health-care providers in DoD, and we are not aware of any recent studies on this topic. Noteworthy, however, is that only the Air Force and Marine Corps made us aware of programs aimed at improving the skills of behavioral health-care providers with respect to assessing and managing suicidal patients. In the Air Force, a sustainment strategy exists that relies on those who have been trained to train new providers during internship and residency programs, providing resources to new providers at local clinics, and through inspections. We were not made aware of a sustainment strategy in the Marine Corps.

Restrict Access to Lethal Means

Across the services, there are no known specific policies in place in which access to lethal means is restricted for the purposes of reducing suicide, either universally or for those at increased or imminent risk of suicide.[2]

Respond Appropriately to Suicides and Suicide Attempts

Although it has yet to be empirically shown to reduce suicides, developing an appropriate response to the aftermath of a suicide is considered a fundamental component of suicide prevention. Each service has a team or personnel on whom leaders can call to assist them after a suicide specifically or traumatic event more generally. However, no policies or guidance provide details on what should be done if and when a unit experiences the loss of one of its own to suicide.

Recommendations

In this section, we provide 14 recommendations pertinent to all services, two of which are overarching recommendations regarding surveillance and evaluation; the remaining 12 are dispersed across each of the six domains that are the key components of effective suicide-prevention programs. Some of our recommendations require the reallocation of additional resources, which will be determined by how DoD and the individual services prioritize our suggestions. When appropriate, we highlight initiatives within DoD that may already be in place attempting to achieve a specific recommendation.

Overarching Recommendations

Recommendation 1: Track Suicides and Suicide Attempts Systematically and Consistently. *Notable programs in DoD: DoDSER.* Each service had a suicide surveillance system in place before 2008, but the recent initiatives to use the DoDSER and establish a common nomenclature across all services are noteworthy. These processes will help ensure that communication about suicide is consistent within DoD. Similarly, through the SPARRC and cross-service military suicide-prevention conference, a consistent nomenclature and surveillance system can help foster information sharing between the services. However, the services currently have different policies regarding DoDSERs for nonfatal behaviors; efforts should be made to ensure consistency across the services in this area.

Recommendation 2: Evaluate Existing Programs and Ensure That New Programs Contain an Evaluation Component When They Are Implemented. *Notable programs*

---

[2] An exception is the Air Force, which provides guidance for leaders in the Leader's Guide for Managing Personel in Distress that, when an airman is suicidal, leaders should "[r]emove all potential means of self-harm from [the airman's] area such as firearms, pills, knives, rope, and machinery." This guide is available on the AFSPP website (U.S. Air Force, undated).

in DoD: AFSPP. This monograph highlights that, to date, very few suicide-prevention programs have been evaluated. While, to some extent, this limits guidance on what programs are most effective, it also positions DoD and each service to contribute to the science by evaluating the programs they have in place to prevent suicide. In fact, DoD and each service are particularly well poised to make a significant contribution to suicide-prevention science because sound evaluations are particularly feasible in the military context due to the large numbers of individuals exposed to prevention programs, long follow-up periods during which outcomes can be assessed and evaluated, and good records, including cause-of-death determinations (at least among those on active duty). These features were integral in evaluating the AFSPP (Knox et al., 2003), which is one of only a handful of suicide-prevention programs listed in the Substance Abuse and Mental Health Service Administration's (SAMHSA's) National Registry of Evidence-Based Programs and Practices (NREPP) (SAMHSA, 2010). Even smaller-scale evaluation efforts, such as pilot studies at research-friendly installations, could make a valuable contribution to preventing suicide in DoD and contribute to the science more generally.

Efforts to evaluate existing suicide-prevention programs and integrate evaluation plans into new initiatives will help ensure that the DoD approach to suicide prevention aligns with the National Strategy for Suicide Prevention (U.S. Public Health Service, 2001), which stresses program evaluation. Evaluation provides a scientific basis for decisionmaking and helps ensure that DoD is performing effectively and can be held accountable for its actions (Milstein and Wetterhall, 1999). While such evaluations would optimally look at the effect of programs on actual suicides, informative evaluations could examine the effects of programs on suicide attempts and ideation as well as referrals to behavioral health care or chaplains. Pre- and posttests delivered before and after training can also provide valuable information on changes in behavior, including intervening on behalf of a peer in distress, and changes in knowledge and attitudes about suicide, mental health, or accessing behavioral health care. They can also be used to ensure that there are not unanticipated or negative effects of the program (Bryan, Dhillon-Davis, and Dhillon-Davis, 2009). Suicide-prevention programs could also be evaluated for cost-effectiveness to ensure that the resources being spent on preventing suicide are achieving anticipated outcomes.

Recommendations for Raising Awareness and Promoting Self-Care

Recommendation 3: Include Training in Skill Building, Particularly Help-Seeking Behavior, in Programs and Initiatives That Raise Awareness and Promote Self-Care. *Notable programs in DoD: Army's ACE seminar-based training; Army's "Beyond the Front" video (Sheftick, 2008).* Within each of the services, universal prevention programs are primarily public awareness campaigns. These campaigns may provide messages about suicide prevention on posters, through videos, and in slide presentations. They generally focus on raising awareness about suicide, recognizing symptoms in others, and providing resources to which a servicemember can turn when he or she or someone he or she knows is feeling suicidal, and may include messages about the importance of peer gatekeepers. Examples of such programs include the community training offered by the Air Force, the Navy's ACT program, and training that front-line supervisors receive in the Marine Corps. A limitation of these programs is that they do not teach the skills servicemembers may need to refer themselves to mental health professionals or chaplains. As reviewed in Chapter Three, the evidence suggests that awareness campaigns that do not teach these skills are not effective ways to prevent suicides.

Two recent suicide-prevention initiatives in the Army are notable exceptions. Although primarily a gatekeeper training program, the ACE campaign includes a three-hour training seminar that includes some skill-building exercises. "Beyond the Front" is an interactive video also sponsored by the Army, in which soldiers viewing the video assume the role of either a soldier who is considering harming himself while deployed or a commander who is concerned about one of his peers. In both cases, viewers watch segments of the video and make decisions that include asking for help and may help build the skills necessary to self-refer, though a formal evaluation of "Beyond the Front" has yet to be conducted.

Although reviewing the DoD programs that promote resiliency was outside of the purview of the current study, the recent shift toward these programs (exemplified by the Army's COSC program and Navy's OSC program) has implications for suicide prevention. Effectively, resiliency programs represent a positive step toward promoting self-care and other protective factors that could eventually reduce suicide. However, the underlying message of these programs is important to consider. With respect to suicide prevention, it is imperative that these programs help servicemembers build the skills necessary to become resilient, and critical among these skills is knowing when and how to ask for help. This approach differs fundamentally from programs and messages that encourage servicemembers to find "inner strengths," which assume that each servicemember already has the skills needed to care for him or herself. Furthermore, some experts we interviewed raised concern that, if not properly worded and phrased, messages about resiliency could reinforce stigma for those with mental health problems or with respect to seeking mental health care if the message conveys the notion that these individuals and behaviors are de facto "weak."

Recommendation 4: Define the Scope of What Is Relevant to Preventing Suicide, and Form Partnerships with the Agencies and Organizations Responsible for Initiatives in Other Areas. *Notable programs in DoD: Air Force's IDS; Navy's OSC; Army's COSC; Marine Corps' informal colocation of prevention initiatives at HQMC; DoD's Real Warriors campaign.* The evidence presented in Chapter Two highlights certain factors that correlate with or increase the risk of suicide. Prominent among these are mental and substance-use disorders, as well as heavy substance use. It was outside the scope of the current study to evaluate DoD-sponsored programs that aim to prevent mental health problems and encourage help-seeking behavior as well as DoD-sponsored substance-use prevention programs. Similarly, it was beyond the scope to evaluate the breadth of services offered by DoD that aim to mitigate negative life events or the effect of such events on individuals' well-being (including, for example, relationship breakups and financial hardship). However, efforts across each of these domains have the potential to affect suicides in DoD. Thus, it is important that suicide-prevention programs within each service create partnerships with the organizations responsible for these areas to ensure consistent messaging, create jointly sponsored projects, and avoid duplication.

The Air Force's IDS is an example of how the Air Force formally established a program to foster such collaboration by means of an Air Force instruction. Although not formalized, the Marine Corps also reports that collaboration across these organizations occurs organically through the colocation of prevention programs on the same floor of the HQMC building, all of which are part of the Marine and Personal and Family Readiness Division.

The Navy's OSC program and Army's COSC program are designed to be comprehensive and are focused on building resilient sailors and soldiers. Such programs may promote protective factors common across many of the psychological or behavioral problems that can eventually lead to suicide. However, it is unclear how these resiliency programs align with the existing agencies and programs geared toward preventing specific psychological or behavioral problems, such as suicide and substance use. Efforts should be made to ensure that these new programs interlock with other prevention programs. In addition, the resiliency programs focus almost solely on promoting protective factors, one of six components of a comprehensive suicide-prevention program. In light of the paucity of research indicating the effectiveness of such programs, care should be taken not to divert too many resources toward these approaches at the expense of programs with some evidence of effectiveness. A wide focus to suicide prevention helps ensure that no servicemember will "fall through the cracks."

Finally, current research efforts are now under way to examine DoD-sponsored programs focused on resiliency and substance-abuse prevention. It will be important for those organizations responsible for suicide prevention to stay abreast of these efforts. Within RAND, at the time of this writing, there were ongoing studies on resiliency run through the RAND Center for Military Health Policy Research. We are also aware of a study to understand substance-abuse prevention programs being conducted by the IOM. A number of other research efforts are also likely under way.

Recommendations for Identifying High-Risk Individuals

Recommendation 5: Evaluate Gatekeeper Training. Given the strong reliance on gatekeeper training in the Army, Navy, and Marines to identify high-risk individuals and the lack of evidence about such programs, evaluating such training programs is particularly important. Though widespread, there are conflicting notions about how effective or ineffective such programs may be. Gatekeeper training might be an effective way to reduce suicide: Peer gatekeepers can reach a wide number of people, while nonmilitary gatekeepers might help reduce the stigma associated with recognizing and referring a peer in uniform. However, having all servicemembers trained to be gatekeepers could possibly send a message that suicide is always another person's problem. Some evidence indicates that, given the same training, not everyone will be equally effective at being a gatekeeper. Also, without clear policies and procedures on the repercussions associated with seeking behavioral health care, servicemembers may not intervene, out of fear that their actions could jeopardize their fellow servicemember's military career. Sound evaluations of these programs are needed to help clarify some of these hypotheses.

Recommendation 6: Develop Prevention Programs Based on Research and Surveillance; Selected and Indicated Programs Should Be Based on Clearly Identified Risk Factors Specific to Military Populations and to Each Service. *Notable programs in DoD: Air Force Investigative Interview Policy; Air Force LPSP program.* Across the services, the majority of reports regarding suicides are case series, which provide descriptive information about servicemembers who have killed themselves. As stated in Chapter Two, while useful, this study design cannot identify the factors that actually place individuals at risk of killing themselves. To identify risk factors, suicide cases must be compared to a well-defined control group. Although the design of the study is at its nascent stage, it is anticipated that the recent collaborative research effort between NIMH and the Army will be helpful in identifying risk factors for suicide within that service.

The identification of risk factors is critical in the development of selected and indicated prevention programs, which are important components of a public health approach to suicide prevention. Across the services, only one notable program stood out in this domain. In developing its suicide-prevention program, the Air Force recognized that airmen under criminal investigation were at increased risk of killing themselves, and two of the 11 tenets that comprise this program are geared specifically to this at-risk group. Under the Investigative Interview Policy, Air Force investigators are required to notify an airman's commander, first sergeant, or supervisor that the airman is under investigation; those airmen appearing emotionally distraught after an interview are released only to a commander, first sergeant, supervisor, or designee. These leaders then assume the responsibility of assessing the airman's emotional state and contact a behavioral health provider if there is an indication of suicidal thoughts. Under the "limited patient privilege" component, from the time of official notification that they are under investigation, airmen become eligible for LPSP, which ensures that information revealed to a mental health provider may not be utilized in a UCMJ action and cannot be used to characterize service at time of separation. However, while, in general, the AFSPP has been shown to be a promising prevention program, the specific tenets of the program, including the Investigative Interview Policy and limited patient privilege policy have not been evaluated.

Research can guide not only who should receive selected and indicated interventions but also the mode in which interventions should be delivered. Emerging evidence suggests that, while in their nascent stage, interventions delivered via the Internet, which includes not only presentation of information online but also mental health screening tools (such as the DoD-funded Military Pathways® program accessible from Military Pathways [undated]), online support groups, online group therapy, or self-directed therapy, can effectively promote mental well-being (Christensen, Griffiths, and Jorm, 2004; Ybarra and Eaton, 2005). There is also evidence to suggest that interventions delivered via mobile telephone short message service (SMS) can effectively create behavior change (Fjeldsoe, Marshall, and Miller, 2009). However, none of these methods has yet been associated with reductions in suicide.

Finally, while interventions designed for civilian populations may be useful benchmarks on which to build prevention programs in the military, care should be taken to adapt programs in recognition of military culture. This means addressing cultural norms and values in the military not only relative to the civilian population but also between services and installations that may themselves each hold different beliefs and values. Also, though rarely investigated, researchers believe that the same intervention may yield different effects across different demographic subgroups, such as between males and females (Leitner, Barr, and Hobby, 2008). Thus, researchers stress that intervention strategies and curriculum, the measures used to evaluate program effectiveness, the length and setting of the intervention, and the manner in which it is delivered may need to be adapted for different groups of individuals (Joe, Canetto, and Romer, 2008).

Recommendation 7: Ensure That Continuity of Service and Care Is Maintained When Servicemembers or Their Caregivers Transition Between Installations in a Process That Respects Servicemembers' Privacy and Autonomy. The Blue Ribbon panel that evaluated suicide-prevention programs in the VHA was cautious in its evaluation of a new procedure that places flags in the electronic medical records of patients assessed for suicidal risk. The intent of the flag is to improve communication between providers about patients' risk status, and it was designed to deal with the increase in suicide risk among patients with mental illness during times of transition. However, caution was expressed that such a flag could increase stigmatization, particularly if these flags are accessible in VHA systems across the country.

Military personnel, including behavioral health-care providers, other caregivers, such as chaplains, and the servicemembers for whom these professionals care, transition frequently. They deploy for significant periods of time; they move between installations and commands; they transition between active and reserve; and they separate from service. Members of the RC, including the National Guard, face additional transitions associated with being placed on active status, training, deploying, returning from deployment, and being placed on nonactive status. It is important that continuity of care is ensured across each of these transition points.

First and foremost, continuity of care across transition points involves ensuring that servicemembers are aware of the resources available in theater, at each new base, and in each new community, as these resources and their location may differ across these areas. For those receiving formal mental health care or informal care from a chaplain, efforts should be made to help ensure that the servicemember continues to receive the care he or she needs, both when he or she transitions and when his or her caregiver leaves one patient population for another. For behavioral health-care providers in particular, managing patients' treatment, particularly their response to prescribed medications, including those prescribed in theater (M. Thompson, 2008), is an important and fundamental component of managing mental illness (Mann, 2005).

To protect the privacy of the servicemember and avoid possible stigmatization, we recommend that processes in place to ensure that servicemembers receive continuity of care be patient-focused in line with the IOM's recommendation of delivering "patient-centered care" (IOM, 2006). Thus, mental health professionals and chaplains should, at a minimum, provide clients moving to a new installation with the contact information for analogous resources at the new installation and encourage their clients to make appointments soon after arriving. If possible and desired, they should arrange appointments prior to the move and obtain permission to transfer records to the new provider so that the new provider is ready to receive the patient and can reach out if appointments are missed. Similarly, these providers should consider following up with clients after they have moved to ensure that they are doing well and that they have maintained the care that they had been receiving prior to the move. If not, this is an ideal time to encourage them to access the necessary resources. A notable policy in the Air Force is AF 41-210 that puts in place procedures for ensuring continuity of care for active outpatient mental health cases, including those being seen at Life Skills Support Centers, Alcohol and Drug Abuse Prevention and Treatment (ADAPT) offices, and the Family Advocacy Office, that are transitioning between installations (AFI 41-210).

Recommendations for Facilitating Access to Quality Care

Recommendation 8: Make Servicemembers Aware of the Benefits of Accessing Behavioral Health Care, Specific Policies and Repercussions for Accessing Such Care, and Conduct Research to Inform This Communication. *Notable programs in DoD: DoD's Real Warriors campaign.* Military personnel share a widespread concern that seeking mental or behavioral health care could harm their career. The recent Real Warriors campaign attempts to address this concern by promoting videos on its website (DCoE, undated) that feature servicemembers revealing that they benefited from behavioral health care and that they did not suffer negative career repercussions. However, although some information on use of behavioral health-care services among servicemembers is collected (for example, as part of the security clearance application),[3] there are no explicit policies with respect to repercussions across the services for accessing behavioral health care. Absent these policies, research is needed to discern the effect that seeking such care has on individuals' military careers. This research would ideally examine whether those who access these services are as likely to attain the same rank as those who do not, as well as differences in the pace at which they advance through ranks (e.g., Rowan and Campise, 2006). However, to ensure valid comparisons, this research should also account for baseline differences between those who access services and those who do not. Ideally, such research would examine differences between three groups: those without mental health symptoms who do not access specialty services, those with mental health symptoms who do access these services, and those with mental health symptoms who do not access these services.

Recommendation 9: Make Servicemembers Aware of the Different Types of Behavioral Health Caregivers Available to Them, Including Information on Caregivers' Credentials, Capabilities, and the Confidentiality Afforded by Each. *Notable programs in DoD: Confidentiality afforded by DoD chaplaincy; Air Force LPSP program.* In 2006, the IOM recognized that the variability in education, licensing, certification, and credentialing in the mental health and substance-use workforce challenges that workforce's capacity to improve or ensure the quality of care offered to those who access it. Without a minimum level of competency across the wide range of professionals who offer behavioral health care, consumers may be unclear about the "safest, most effective, and most efficient care" for their unique needs (IOM, 2006). The military represents a microcosm of this workforce that includes "psychologists, psychiatrists, other specialty or primary care physicians, social workers, psychiatric nurses, marriage and family therapists, addiction therapists, psychosocial rehabilitation therapists, sociologists, and a variety of counselors with different education and certifications" (IOM, 2006). Each service also relies heavily on chaplains who are embedded in military units and often serve as front-line responders for persons under psychological or emotional duress.

In the general community and across services, there is variety in the unique attributes and offerings of each of these professions, described in detail in the IOM report (2006). Educating military personnel about the differences across referral endpoints with respect to each professional's credentials and capabilities is important. Since peer-focused gatekeeper training often highlights these organizations and personnel as referral endpoints, including descriptions of each in this setting would be helpful. However, it is just as, if not more, important for providers of each type to know what kind of care they are capable of providing and refer as appropriate.

---

[3]   In May 2008, the wording of the question on prior mental health consultation was changed to exclude counseling strictly for combat stress or related to marital, family, or grief issues.

In the military specifically, confidentiality, which is noted to be a specific barrier to care among this population, is not uniform. Chaplains offer total confidentiality and are not supposed to divulge any information to command staff or others about who has accessed their services or what they have said in counseling sessions (though they may begin sessions with a disclaimer allowing them permission to report specific cases, such as child or spouse abuse) (Barry, 2003). On the other hand, command staff have access to information about servicemembers' access of professional mental health services (i.e., care offered in a clinical setting), which may influence an individual's decision to seek this type of care. Steps for improving confidentiality are discussed in detail elsewhere (Tanielian et al., 2008).

Recommendation 10: Improve Coordination and Communication Between Caregivers and Service Providers. *Notable programs in DoD: Air Force's IDS.* Behavioral health-care providers in the military include psychiatrists, psychologists, nurses, counselors, chaplains, and primary-care physicians. These professionals should work as a team to ensure that the emotional well-being of those for whom they care is maintained. We heard disparate reports about the relationship among these professionals on military bases. For example, some interviewees reported very open communication and collegiality between chaplains and behavioral health-care providers, and others reported a more acrimonious relationship. To the extent that some of these professionals actually serve as gatekeepers, improved communication and collaboration between professionals helps create a trustworthy hand-off to ensure that individuals do not fall through the cracks when going from one form of care to another.

One noteworthy initiative that helps foster communication between these different entities is the Air Force's installation-level IDS, which coordinates the prevention missions of chaplains, child and youth programs, Family Advocacy, Family Support, Health Promotion/Health and Wellness Centers, and mental health clinics. The IDS is intended to develop a comprehensive and coordinated plan for integrating community outreach and prevention programs, including suicide prevention, and to eliminate duplication, overlap, and gaps in delivering prevention services by consolidating existing committees with similar charters.

Recommendation 11: Assess Whether There Is an Adequate Supply of Behavioral Health-Care Professionals and Chaplains Available to Servicemembers. Whether through the use of gatekeeper programs or through programs that encourage self-referral, effective suicide prevention in the military will rely on persons accessing quality behavioral health care and counseling services. Such messages assume a capacity of providers and chaplains who can deliver quality care and counseling to those who request it. It was beyond the scope of the current project to assess the workforce capacity of behavioral health-care professionals and chaplains, but there appears to be a need for research to address this concern. Chaplains, for example, reported that they thought they were understaffed, though they did not have an empirical basis for this assumption. There is a known shortage of behavioral health professionals in the United

States generally, and DoD has faced challenges in recruiting and retaining adequately trained behavioral health professionals (Burnam et al., 2008). It is a disservice to refer people to behavioral health care or tell them about the benefits of such services when appointments are not readily available for them.

Recommendations for Providing Quality Care

Recommendation 12: Mandate Training on Evidence-Based or State-of-the-Art Practices for Behavioral Health Generally and in Suicide Risk Assessment and Management Specifically for Chaplains, Health-Care Providers, and Behavioral Health-Care Professionals. *Notable programs in DoD: Air Force/Marine one-time training, ASIST, RESPECT-Mil.* Not only do programs that promote using behavioral health professionals and chaplains operate under the assumption that there is sufficient capacity of these professionals available, but they also assume that all of those to whom they refer individuals in crisis are sufficiently trained in assessing and managing suicidal patients. Unfortunately, this assumption is not sound: Few providers are adequately trained on effective ways to assess risk and manage patients at varying levels of risk, possibly due to the paucity of research linking assessment and treatment techniques to reductions in actual suicides (see Chapter Three). Nonetheless, guides do exist that, while not evidence-based, offer helpful guidelines to providers. Within the military, both the Air Force and Marine Corps have independently trained behavioral health-care providers on guidelines for managing and providing care for suicidal individuals. The Air Force contracted these training programs to the SPRC; the current Marine Corps SPPM is trained to deliver SPRC's in-house training, "Assessing and Managing Suicide Risk," and, over the course of a year, visited Marine Corps bases to offer the training. However, both of these training initiatives were one-time initiatives, and there is no plan to offer similar training in the future. In addition, the training sessions were voluntary but could be made mandatory.

Above and beyond the assumption that health-care providers are trained specifically in managing and assessment of suicidal behaviors is an implicit assumption that these professionals are trained to provide high-quality care. Unfortunately, research from the civilian sector indicates that the provision of quality care for behavioral health care is not universal across behavioral health-care providers (IOM, 2006), and there is no reason to think that services in the military are any different. The quality of mental health care offered in DoD is unknown, and efforts to improve quality, such as training providers in evidence-based practice, are not integrated into the system of care (Burnam et al., 2008). Again, recommendations to improve the quality of mental health care offered in DoD treatment facilities is offered elsewhere (Tanielian et al., 2008) and may include training providers to deliver evidence-based care and reimbursing only those services that are deemed to be evidence-based.

Ensuring quality of care will also require vigilant overview of the science developing in this area that may have implications for suicide prevention in the military.

Promising advances for mental health treatment that may eventually reduce suicidal behaviors include emerging pharmacotherapy and psychotherapies aimed at depression and PTSD. In addition, DoD should stay abreast of advances in telehealth technology, particularly with respect to ways in which providers can use Internet-based applications to provide patient-centered care (Christensen, Griffiths, and Jorm, 2004; Litz et al., 2007; Ybarra and Eaton, 2005).

Two other programs are worth noting in promoting improved care for mental health issues in the Army. First, specific to suicide, chaplains in the Army and in the Air Force are offered ASIST, a two-day workshop geared toward teaching first responders the tools necessary for managing a person in imminent risk of harming him or herself. Second, the Army Surgeon General has disseminated the RESPECT-Mil treatment program to selected Army primary-care facilities. RESPECT-Mil is designed to promote screening, assessment, treatment, and referral among Army soldiers presenting to primary-care facilities with depression or PTSD.

Recommendations for Restricting Access to Lethal Means

Recommendation 13: Develop Creative Strategies to Restrict Access to Lethal Means Among Military Servicemembers or Those Indicated to Be at Risk of Harming Themselves. A comprehensive suicide-prevention strategy should have considered ways to restrict access to lethal means that servicemembers could use to take their own lives. This includes the use of blister packs for lethal medications to prevent intentional overdoses, bridge safeguards to prevent fatal falls, and constructing shower-curtain rods so as to prevent fatal hangings. Additionally, due to the prevalence of firearms as a means by which military servicemembers kill themselves, initiatives to restrict access to firearms should be considered.

Although restricting firearms among those specifically trained to use them and for whom the use of firearms may be a function of their job seems daunting or even impossible, there is precedent for such policies, both in the VHA and in DoD. In particular, selected or indicated prevention strategies may include restricting access to firearms among those identified to be at risk of harming themselves. One recent study in the VHA, for example, found that suicidal patients relied primarily on family members to restrict their access to firearms during times of suicidal crises but that such patients found it acceptable for clinicians to ask about firearm ownership, distribute trigger locks, and even provide safe offsite storage of firearms (Roeder et al., 2009). The 1996 Lautenberg amendment (Pub. L. 104-208 §658) to the Gun Control Act of 1968 (Pub. L. 90-618) restricts those convicted of a misdemeanor domestic-violence offense to ship, transport, possess, or receive firearms and ammunition. This rule applies to military personnel as well and to firearms and ammunition used for either personal or professional purposes.

Recommendations for Responding Appropriately

Recommendation 14: Provide Formal Guidance to Commanders About How to Respond to Suicides and Suicide Attempts. *Notable programs in DoD: Air Force's TSR; Navy's SPRINT and CACOs; New Hampshire Army National Guard.* Responding to a suicide appropriately not only can help acquaintances of the suicide victim grieve but also can prevent possible imitative suicides and interrupt possible suicide clusters, as well as serve as a conduit to care for those at high risk. It is noteworthy that each of the services has crisis response teams to help military units and installations deal with a traumatic event, including a suicide. However, the effectiveness of some crisis response approaches is controversial. For example, the evidence does not support single-session "debriefings" after a traumatic or critical event as being effective at reducing psychological distress, and, in a few trials, such debriefings even appear to be detrimental (Rose et al., 2002). Across services, there is no direct policy or guidance regarding appropriate ways in which a leader should respond to a suicide within his or her unit, including how to talk to the media about suicides and how military-sponsored media cover these events. Fear of imitative suicides may also hinder many leaders from openly discussing suicides in their units.

In 1988, the CDC provided recommendations for a "community plan for the prevention and containment of suicide clusters" (O'Carroll, Mercy, and Steward, 1988). It outlined a plan that is community-specific and built around bringing responsible organizations, agencies, and community leaders together to align roles and responsibilities and to implement a coordinated response. Results from at least one case study suggest that such an approach may have successfully contained or contributed to the containment of a possible suicide contagion (Hacker et al., 2008). The New Hampshire Army National Guard has partnered with New Hampshire NAMI to apply a similar approach to respond to suicides in that organization. The CONNECT model is a postvention program that brings key stakeholders (e.g., law enforcement, medical examiners, clergy) together to develop a coordinated response to a suicide, with written protocols clearly defining stakeholders' roles and responsibilities in the event of a suicide. Particularly noteworthy is that the program also recommends establishing a template script before a suicide so that military leaders know how to communicate information while minimizing the possibility of imitation.

Although not considered postvention per se, there also needs to be guidance for leaders to help care for and integrate servicemembers back into units after those servicemembers have made suicide attempts or expressed suicidal ideation. There are many anecdotal reports of servicemembers being ostracized or ridiculed after seeking mental health care or having been treated for suicidal behavior. Not only does this increase the risk of another suicide attempt, but it also creates a hostile and stigmatizing environment for others in the unit who may be under psychological or emotional duress.

Final Thoughts

Suicide is a tragic event, and, although evidence is scant, comments from the experts we interviewed, in addition to the literature we reviewed, suggest that it can be prevented. The military has in place many programs that aim to prevent suicide, though the number of suicides that it has actually prevented is inestimable. The recommendations we provide represent the ways in which the best available evidence suggests that even more of these untimely deaths could be avoided.

Appendixes

The appendixes contain a brief description of the suicide-prevention programs and initiatives across each service: the Army (Appendix A), Navy (Appendix B), Air Force (Appendix C), and Marine Corps (Appendix D). Initiatives included in these lists meet three criteria:

1. The initiative *targets active-duty military* and/or military personnel who have recently been deployed. Initiatives for families and civilian workers employed by the specific service are not included.
2. The initiative's *primary purpose is to prevent suicide.* This means that the initiative was designed to directly influence suicidal behavior. Initiatives that may indirectly prevent suicide by targeting a known risk factor were not included. For example, substance abuse is a risk factor associated with suicidal behavior. However, substance-abuse prevention and counseling programs were not included in this document because substance-abuse prevention—not suicide prevention—is the primary purpose of these programs.
3. The initiative is *run by the specific service.* Service personnel are involved in the planning and implementation of the initiative and control the funding for the initiative.

Army Suicide-Prevention Initiatives

Table A.1
Army Suicide Prevention Program

Feature	Description
Brief description	The omnibus ASPP is run by the Army G-1, through DAPE-HRI.
Target outcomes	The goal of the ASPP is to minimize suicidal behavior among soldiers, family members, DA civilians, and retirees. Five overarching strategies are used to accomplish this: - develop positive life coping skills - encourage help-seeking behavior - raise awareness of and vigilance toward suicide prevention - synchronize, integrate, and manage the ASPP - conduct suicide surveillance, analysis, and reporting.
Target population	Active-duty soldiers, RC, ARNG, and Army civilians
Setting/scope of initiative	The ASPP focuses on maintaining the individual readiness of the soldier and civilian. This is accomplished through the Army Suicide Prevention Model, which contains prevention (main effort), intervention, and postvention materials.
Implementation history	The ASPP began in 1984.
Initiative costs or resource requirements	No cost data are available, as the current ASPP is not a program of record.
Evaluation design and outcomes	None available
IOM category	Universal
Published information	The program is represented on the G-1's website, at http://www.armyg1.army.mil/hr/suicide/default.asp (as of March 30, 2010). Policies, roles, and responsibilities of the ASPP are contained in Army doctrine: AR 600-63 and DA PAM 600-24.
Managing office	Office of the Deputy Chief of Staff, G-1 DAPE-HRI (Suicide Prevention) ATTN: The Army SPPM (as of July 2004, the SPPM was Walter Morales, walter.morales@hqda.army.mil)

NOTE: ARNG = Army National Guard.

Table A.2
Three-Part Training

Feature	Description
Brief description	In March 2009, the Army unveiled what is often referred to as a "three-part training" program to bolster its suicide-prevention programs. The first part ("stand down") included an interactive video called "Beyond the Front," along with materials from the ACE program. The second part ("chain teach") contains the "Shoulder to Shoulder" video and a suicide-prevention training tip card intended to augment the first part with a more deliberate and personal approach. The third part is annual training using existing suicide-prevention training resources.
Target outcomes	Soldiers, leaders and commanders at all levels, DA civilians, and family members - understand suicide risk factors - recognize warning signs - learn how to intervene and take appropriate intervention actions as warranted - reduce suicidal behavior across the Army as a result.
Target population	Army-wide but focused on soldiers, leaders, Army families, and DA civilians
Setting and scope of initiative	Training is provided through supervisors and leaders within military units and establishments.
Implementation history	With increasing suicide rates, the Army Chief of Staff ordered a stand-down followed by a deliberate chain-teaching program focused on suicide prevention. The stand-down was ordered for all DA civilians, soldiers, and family members and was to be completed between February 15, 2009, and March 15, 2009. The chain teaching was to be completed between March 15, 2009, and July 15, 2009. Phase 3 was initiated at phase 1 (i.e., they run parallel, not sequentially) and continues ad infinitum with sustainment teaching.
Initiative costs or resource requirements	Teaching and training materials are available to all soldiers through AKO and elsewhere. Leaders at all echelons are responsible for implementing the teaching within their units and groups.
Evaluation design and outcomes	None available
IOM category	Universal
Published information	EXORD 103-09 initiated the stand-down and chain-teach portions of the three-part training.
Managing office	Office of the Deputy Chief of Staff, G-1 DAPE-HRI (Suicide Prevention) ATTN: The Army SPPM (as of July 2004, the SPPM was Walter Morales, walter.morales@hqda.army.mil)

NOTE: AKO = Army Knowledge Online. EXORD = executive order.

Table A.3
Strong Bonds

Feature	Description
Brief description	Strong Bonds is a chaplain-led initiative that creates opportunities during weekend retreats for military couples, singles, and families to interact with others who share similar deployment cycles. These groups gather at events to share their experiences and learn of community resources that can help them in times of crisis. While the official information released by the program does not specifically mention suicide prevention, discussions with officials indicate that suicide prevention is part of the impetus of the program. It is a holistic, preventive program committed to the restoration and preservation of Army families.
Target outcomes	- Create a resilient soldier. - Teach relationship-building skills. - Connect soldiers to community health and support resources.
Target population	The program is implemented at the unit level for active-duty, National Guard, and Army Reserve soldiers. Participants are admitted on a first-come, first-serve basis, though recently there have been ongoing efforts to prioritize soldiers who have recently returned or are about to deploy.
Setting and scope of initiative	Strong Bonds is not meant to treat those in crisis, but rather is there to build relationships and communication skills to prevent future problems.
Implementation history	Strong Bonds grew out of a program in the late 1990s called "Building Strong and Ready Families," which was originally formed to combat a rash of divorces within the 25th Infantry Division in Hawaii. In FY 2008, approximately 16,000 personnel (active and reserve) were involved in about 1,800 Strong Bonds events.
Initiative costs or resource requirements	Costs cover advertising, a DVD used within the National Guard, and funds to pay for the weekends away. Previous funding was included in the supplemental budget. More recently, the program has been added as a defense budget line item within the CSF program.
Evaluation design and outcomes	Multiple evaluations ongoing through universities
IOM category	Universal
Published information	Information on Strong Bonds can be found at http://www.strongbonds.org.
Managing office	National Guard Bureau Readiness Center ATTN: Strong Bonds Program Manager

Table A.4
Ask, Care, Escort

Feature	Description
Brief description	ACE is the centerpiece of a new Army-wide suicide intervention skill-training curriculum that targets at-risk soldiers through peer-led interventions. The ACE program includes training information in DVDs, PowerPoint® files, handouts, and training tip cards (wallet cards) accessible through the web to help soldiers identify and assist fellow soldiers at risk for suicide.
Target outcomes	Overall, the goal is to prevent suicides in the Army. More specifically, ACE aims to - teach soldiers how to recognize suicidal behavior in fellow soldiers and the warning signs that accompany it - target soldiers at risk for suicide who are unlikely to seek help due to stigma - increase a soldier's confidence to ask whether a battle buddy is thinking of suicide - teach soldiers skills in active listening - encourage soldiers to take a battle buddy directly to the chain of command, chaplain, or behavioral health provider.
Target population	First-line leaders, battle buddies, Army family members, and civilians
Setting and scope of initiative	ACE is provided at all levels of the Army.
Implementation history	The ACE program was developed within CHPPM and deployed through the Army G-1 ASPP.
Initiative costs or resource requirements	Advertising and materials were developed with internal funds in CHPPM. The ACE program training is meant to take 3 hours and be administered at the platoon level.
Evaluation design and outcomes	Listed in Section III (Adherence to Standards) of the SPRC/AFSP Best Practices Registry, meaning that it addresses specific goals of the *National Strategy for Suicide Prevention* and has been reviewed by a panel of three suicide-prevention experts and found to meet standards of accuracy, safety, and programmatic guidelines. Practices were not reviewed for evidence of effectiveness.
IOM category	Universal
Published information	http://www.sprc.org/featured_resources/bpr/PDF/ArmyACESuicidePreventionProgram.pdf
Managing office	USACHPPM, MCHB-TS-HBH ACE Suicide Intervention Program Coordinator Email: DHPWWebContacts2@amedd.army.mil

Table A.5
Resiliency Training (formerly Battlemind)

Feature	Description
Brief description	Resiliency training is a compendium of information provided to soldiers on the web in order "to prepare Warriors mentally for the rigors of combat and other military deployments." The information is focused largely on what soldiers can expect to experience once deployed and how to transition once returned. The curriculum focuses on short, pointed, and factual representations of combat in order to facilitate good mental health. Suicide prevention is not directly addressed in resiliency training.
Target outcomes	- Increase soldiers' mental preparedness for the rigors of combat and other military deployments. - Reduce posttraumatic stress symptoms, depression symptoms, sleep problems, and stigma.
Target population	Soldiers, Army leaders, Army family members, and DA civilians. Both pre- and postdeployment modules are available.
Setting and scope of initiative	The training products are developed and tested by the WRAIR and refined by the WRAIR's Battlemind Transition Office. Training support packages are completed by the AMEDD center and school's Battlemind Training Office.
Implementation history	In 2007, Battlemind was mandated as an Army-wide effort. It now resides within the G-3's CSF program as resiliency training.
Initiative costs or resource requirements	WRAIR Division of Psychiatry and Neuroscience developed the program with a budget of approximately $1.2 million. The proponency for Battlemind resides at Fort Sam Houston with a separate budget.
Evaluation design and outcomes	Three randomized controlled studies showed that Battlemind postdeployment training reduced reports of the following for the 4–6 months after training: - PTSD symptoms - depression symptoms - sleeping problems - anger problems - stigma surrounding mental health treatment. Additional studies evaluated Battlemind predeployment training: The MHAT V report from 2007 found that soldiers who received predeployment Battlemind training reported fewer mental health symptoms in theater than those who did not. Other trials are ongoing.
IOM category	Selected or indicated
Published information	http://www.resilience.army.mil
Managing office	Division of Psychiatry and Neuroscience Walter Reed Army Institute of Research

NOTE: WRAIR = Walter Reed Army Institute of Research.

Table A.6
Applied Suicide Intervention Skills Training

Feature	Description
Brief description	ASIST is a training package for installation gatekeepers to help those experiencing suicidal thoughts and those trying to assist those in crisis. The training does not produce qualified personnel to diagnose mental disorders or directly treat individuals, but rather provides intervention training for gatekeepers and "green tab" leaders.
Target outcomes	- Identify soldiers who have thoughts of suicide. - Understand how gatekeepers' beliefs and attitudes can affect suicide intervention. - Seek a shared understanding of the reasons for thoughts of suicide and the reasons for living. - Assess current risk and develop a plan to increase safety from suicidal behavior for an agreed amount of time. - Follow up on all safety commitments and determine whether additional help is needed.
Target population	The Army's suicide-prevention policy requires at least two ASIST-trained representatives per installation, camp, state, territory, and Reserve Support Center. In addition, all chaplains and their assistants, behavioral health professionals, and Army Community Service staff members must attend the training. Since 2001, thousands of ASIST kits have been distributed Army-wide to support suicide intervention skills training. The Air Force also employs some ASIST packages.
Setting and scope of initiative	The ASIST package focuses on training gatekeepers to identify those around them who might be suicidal. It is meant to teach both professionals and nonprofessionals what is often referred to as "suicide first-aid"—how to identify and respond to someone needing help.
Implementation history	ASIST was developed in the early 1980s at the University of Calgary in Alberta, Canada, and a decade later was the basis for the company Living Works Education. The ASIST package is marketed around the world under various names.
Initiative costs or resource requirements	Not available
Evaluation design and outcomes	- The Kirkpatrick model (consisting of a literature review; an analysis of the national ASIST database; a national online survey; interviews and focus groups with national and local stakeholders, ASIST trainers, and participants; and in-depth local implementation studies (LISs) in six selected areas) was used in *The Use and Impact of Applied Suicide Intervention Skills Training (ASIST) in Scotland: An Evaluation* (Griesbach, 2008) - *Evaluation of Applied Suicide Intervention Skills Training (ASIST): West Dunbartonshire* (AskClyde, 2007) - *Gatekeepers: Helping to Prevent Suicide in Colorado* (Colorado Trust, 2007) - *Evaluation of Statewide Training in Student Suicide Prevention* (Williams, Hague, and Cornell, undated) - "Making it Safer: A Health Centre's Strategy for Suicide Prevention" (McAuliffe and Perry, 2007).
IOM category	Selected or indicated
Published information	Information on ASIST can be found at http://www.livingworks.net/AS.php.
Managing office	Living Works Email: usa@livingworks.net Website: http://www.livingworks.net

Table A.7
G-1 Suicide-Prevention Website

Feature	Description
Brief description	The G-1 suicide-prevention website provides access to materials on suicide prevention for soldiers, leaders, trainers, and others. This access includes posters, pamphlets, briefings, videos, training materials, hotlines, and links to other material.
Target outcomes	- Promote awareness of suicide prevention and provide access to prevention programs and resources. - Reduce stigma of accessing mental health resources or care.
Target population	The G-1 site is widely accessible but geared toward soldiers, Army leaders, their families, and DA civilians.
Setting and scope of initiative	The website is available to a wide audience on the web and is periodically updated with new content.
Implementation history	The G-1 suicide-prevention website was established in 2001.
Initiative costs or resource requirements	Unclear
Evaluation design and outcomes	None
IOM category	Universal
Published information	http://www.armyg1.army.mil/hr/suicide/default.asp
Managing office	Office of the Deputy Chief of Staff, G-1 DAPE-HRI (Suicide Prevention) ATTN: The Army SPPM (as of July 2004, the SPPM was Walter Morales, walter.morales@hqda.army.mil)

Table A.8
Warrior Adventure Quest

Feature	Description
Brief description	Provide high-adventure, outdoor activities (such as rafting, skydiving, and rock climbing) to help soldiers returning from combat adjust to life out of theater. The program also offers resiliency training. Suicide prevention is not a specific goal of WAQ, though it is sometimes mentioned along with the program.
Target outcomes	- Reduce fatalities from high-risk activities. - Reduce behavioral incidents. - Increase retention. - Increase other MWR activities.
Target population	Returning soldiers. Planning is under way to bring the program to an additional 24 Army garrisons in 2010, and the long-term goal is to have every Basic Combat Training participant in WAQ within 90 days of redeployment from theater.
Setting and scope of initiative	Following on high rates of injuries and potentially injurious events (e.g., car accidents) experienced by recently returned veterans, this program aims to better acquaint the soldiers with exciting activities as a surrogate for other more dangerous endeavors.
Implementation history	Not available
Initiative costs or resource requirements	WAQ is centrally funded through MWR, with oversight from the Installation Management Command and regional MWR recreation managers. At the time of this writing, the Army was planning to put approximately 80,000 soldiers through WAQ, to which it allocated $7 million.
Evaluation design and outcomes	There are plans to evaluate the program through surveys.
IOM category	Selected or indicated
Published information	Not available
Managing office	MWR Command

NOTE: WAQ = Warrior Adventure Quest. MWR = Family and Morale, Welfare and Recreation Command.

Table A.9
Re-Engineering Systems of Primary Care Treatment in the Military (RESPECT-Mil)

Feature	Description
Brief description	RESPECT-Mil provides primary care–based screening, assessment, treatment, and referral of soldiers with depression and PTSD. It is administered by the Army Surgeon General. RESPECT-Mil does not directly cite suicide prevention as a goal.
Target outcomes	Improve primary-care clinics' detection and treatment of depression and PTSD within the Army.
Target population	AMEDD has adopted RESPECT-Mil and, as of this writing, was in place in 15 Army MTFs representing 42 primary-care clinics. TRICARE is in the process of adopting the program.
Setting and scope of initiative	RESPECT-Mil is a treatment model deployed by the Army. It focuses on primary-care providers assisted by trained individuals to screen for depression and PTSD.
Implementation history	RESPECT-Mil originated within the Office of the Army Surgeon General in early 2007. It built on work by three universities (Duke University, Dartmouth College, and Indiana University) through funding from the John D. and Catherine T. MacArthur Foundation.
Initiative costs or resource requirements	Not available
Evaluation design and outcomes	NQMP has been tasked to evaluate the program. See "RESPECT-Mil: Feasibility of a Systems-Level Collaborative Care Approach to Depression and Post-Traumatic Stress Disorder in Military Primary Care" (Engel et al., 2008). Another similar evaluation is "Care Management for Depression in Primary Care Practice: Findings from the RESPECT-Depression Trial" (Nutting et al., 2008).
IOM category	Universal
Published information	http://www.pdhealth.mil/respect-mil/index1.asp
Managing office	Not available

NOTE: NQMP = National Quality Management Program.

Table A.10
The Army Suicide Prevention Task Force

Feature	Description
Brief description	The ASPTF was set up in early 2009 to analyze existing health-promotion systems and processes within the Army and provide recommendations to immediately improve health, reduce risk, and prevent suicides.
Target outcomes	- Reduce suicides within the Army. - Produce an "Army Campaign Plan for Health Promotion, Risk Reduction and Suicide Prevention" (Chiarelli, 2009).
Target population	Army soldiers, DA civilians, and families
Setting and scope of initiative	The ASPTF was an HQDA-level, interim organization, designed to provide immediate, coordinated reporting and programmatic solutions.
Implementation history	At the direction of the Vice Chief of Staff of the Army, the task force was stood up in early 2009.
Initiative costs or resource requirements	Not available
Evaluation design and outcomes	The ASPTF may be dissolved based on retirement of critical tasks from the synchronization matrix, feedback from the field, and substantial subsuming of management by proponent staff and agencies.
IOM category	Universal
Published information	The ASPTF produced three items: - "Army Campaign Plan for Health Promotion, Risk Reduction and Suicide Prevention" (Chiarelli, 2009) - Annex D to the campaign plan, which contains checklists for installation, garrison, and MTF commanders - a synchronization matrix of DOTMLPF actions and responsible organizations.
Managing office	Army Suicide Prevention Task Force Pentagon, 3B548

Table A.11
Comprehensive Soldier Fitness Program

Feature	Description
Brief description	The CSF program works across the physical, emotional, social, spiritual, and family dimensions by taking a holistic approach to fitness, enhancing the performance and resilience of the force. This occurs through assessments, training and education, analysis, and feedback. The CSF program does not explicitly state suicide prevention as a goal.
Target outcomes	- Enhance soldier/family/Army civilian performance and resiliency. - Improve unit readiness and effectiveness. - Change cultural understanding of fitness to include family, emotional, social, and spiritual dimensions. - Implement strategy that assesses and improves comprehensive fitness across institutional, operational, and self-development training throughout all DOTMLPF domains.
Target population	Army, DA civilians, and families
Setting and scope of initiative	With current operational tempo, the Army has recognized a gap in services. Specifically, the Army has identified that it has not - incorporated psychological, emotional, spiritual, and social dimensions of wellness or fitness - trained soldiers in resilience, life skills, and coping strategies - linked programs and interventions with soldiers and families - taught and validated posttraumatic growth.
Implementation history	Established October 1, 2008, as a directorate within the Army G-3/5/7.
Initiative costs or resource requirements	Not available
Evaluation design and outcomes	None
IOM category	Universal
Published information	http://www.army.mil/csf/ (U.S. Army, undated) contains information on the program.
Managing office	G-3/5/7, DAMO-CSF

Table A.12
Mental Health Advisory Teams

Feature	Description
Brief description	MHATs have been deployed to theater to assess the mental and behavioral health of deployed soldiers, the quality of mental and behavioral health care, and access to this care and to make recommendations for changes to improve mental health and mental health services. Since 2003, the OTSG has deployed six MHATs.
Target outcomes	- Assess the mental health of deployed forces. - Examine the delivery of behavioral health care. - Provide recommendations.
Target population	Deployed soldiers, DA civilians, and marines
Setting and scope of initiative	Deployed teams of mental health practitioners conduct interviews, surveys, focus groups, and observation of soldiers and health-care providers in theater. Teams are from WRAIR and subordinate units.
Implementation history	MHATs were initiated in late July 2003 with the support of the Army Surgeon General and Army G-1 in response to an increase in suicides, behavioral health patient flow, and stress and behavioral health issues in Iraq and other deployment locations.
Initiative costs or resource requirements	Not available
Evaluation design and outcomes	Not available
IOM category	Selected or indicated
Published information	Reports and highlights of each MHAT are available at http://www.armymedicine.army.mil/reports/mhat/mhat.html
Managing office	OTSG

NOTE: OTSG = Office of the Surgeon General.

Navy Suicide-Prevention Initiatives

Table B.1
Annual Suicide-Prevention Awareness Training

Feature	Description
Brief description	The annual suicide-prevention awareness training is a GMT given to all sailors through a standardized PowerPoint presentation. A facilitator's guide accompanies the PowerPoint presentation, which includes tips, checklists, and directions for facilitators to conduct activities relevant to the presentation. The training is intended to provide all sailors with the knowledge and action strategies needed to understand and recognize suicidal risk among their peers. The following topics are covered during the training: risk and protective factors, warning signs, the ACT first-responder process, and other relevant suicide resources.
Target outcomes	- All sailors can identify risk factors, protective factors, and warning signs for suicide. - All sailors know to respond, get assistance, identify local resources, and know the acronym ACT.
Target population	All active-duty sailors
Setting and scope of initiative	All sailors are required by OPNAVINST 1720.4A to receive suicide awareness training at least annually.
Implementation history	NETC works with the Navy's Health and Wellness Promotion Program to develop standard content for a GMT module available electronically via the NKO website (NETC, undated). The training is supplemented with information on local procedures and resources. Across the Navy, sailors receive this training in various formats, including online and through presentations by members of their command, chaplains, and FFSC educators and counselors (upon command request). Commands are encouraged to invite support personnel to their training to familiarize sailors with chaplains and FFSC staff.
Initiative costs or resource requirements	NETC staff time is devoted to periodically updating the online training module and integrating local procedures and resources into the training. In addition, all sailors must be given time to attend the training.
Evaluation design and outcomes	NKO module includes a learning assessment. The Behavioral Health Quick Poll (Newell, Whittam, and Uriell, 2009) assessed overall compliance, self-efficacy, and knowledge.
IOM category	Universal
Published information	None available
Managing office	Education and Training Command, U.S. Navy https://www.netc.navy.mil/ NKO website: https://wwwa.nko.navy.mil/portal/home/

NOTE: NKO = Navy Knowledge Online.

Table B.2
Leadership Messages and Newsletters About Suicide Prevention

Feature	Description
Brief description	The naval communication plan outlines communication strategy about suicide awareness. This includes messages and newsletters from senior leadership (e.g., generals, commanders) emphasizing suicide awareness and behavioral health–related topics. Examples of types of communication include Rhumb Lines, Anchor Lines, Daily News Update newscasts, Captain's Call Kit, POD notes, and a variety of others. NMCPHC and Navy Safety Center also assist in communicating suicide-prevention information. The primary messages communicated are as follows: - Life counts, live it. - What sailors do makes a difference to their shipmates and the Navy. - Using support resources in a timely way is a sign of strength and a duty to stay mission ready. - Sailors should reach out for help. Shipmates should look out for each other: An officer/sailor in crisis may not be able to reach out for help, so it is up to someone on the outside to intervene. - Sailors should practice the ACT model to help fellow sailors.
Target outcomes	Improve awareness among sailors about the signs and symptoms of suicide and available resources
Target population	All active-duty sailors
Setting and scope of initiative	The communications are delivered through a variety of media: - Poster series: There are currently a series of four suicide-prevention posters available online and for order from the Naval Logistic Library. Multiple copies of each are also distributed to each installation for display in high-traffic areas, such as a gas station, commissary, or gym. Posters are rotated bimonthly. - Brochures: A suicide-prevention brochure is available both online and at FFSCs. - Websites: The Navy launched a suicide-specific URL for its suicide-prevention website to promote suicide-prevention awareness. Suicide-prevention materials are also available through a variety of other departments of the Navy, including the Deployment Health Unit, NETC, and BUMED. - Newsletters and emails: Articles and announcements about the signs and symptoms of suicide and available resources are published regularly in a variety of newsletters. - Videos: Both PSAs and informational videos that address the signs and symptoms of suicide are available. PSAs are shown on the Navy television channel, while informational videos are available online or on DVD by request. - Radio spots: Suicide-prevention messages are also communicated through the Direct-to-Sailor radio station.
Implementation history	A new http://www.suicide.navy.mil URL (NAVPERS, 2010a) went live in September 2008. A sailor suggested the new address after he discovered that his sailor son had searched online for "suicide" and "suicide+navy" in the weeks before attempting suicide in January 2008. A new four-poster series was distributed to all installations in November 2008 along with a new trifold brochure. A family-targeted suicide-prevention brochure was planned for FY 2009. In July 2009, a suicide-prevention poster contest was sponsored by the Navy's Behavioral Health Department. The winner's poster will be distributed Navy-wide and featured in the All Hands magazine. One new video on suicide prevention was planned for release in fall 2009. A postvention video and a video targeted for providers are being edited for release in FY 2010.

Table B.2—Continued

Feature	Description
Initiative costs or resource requirements	Unknown, multiple units and budgets support these activities.
Evaluation design and outcomes	Some metrics of communication effort are monitored, such as visits to the suicide.navy.mil website.
IOM Category	Universal
Published information	The suicide-prevention brochure, posters, and videos are available online at http://www.suicide.navy.mil.
Managing office	Navy Personnel Command http://www.npc.navy.mil

NOTE: POD = plan of the day.

Table B.3
Reserve Psychological Health Outreach Program

Feature	Description
Brief description	The Reserve Psychological Health Outreach Program provides (1) psychological health education that includes the Operational Stress Control Awareness's suicide-prevention component; (2) initial clinical assessments of redeployed reservists' mental health and appropriate care referral; and (3) psychological health assessments requested by reserve units for members affected by suicides or suicide attempts.
Target outcomes	- Identify reservists with mental health needs. - Work on a more dedicated basis with reservists with mental health needs to ensure that they receive appropriate care. - Mitigate the impact of a suicide completion or attempt on reservist units.
Target population	All reservists in the Navy
Setting and scope of initiative	All the activities conducted through this program take place at the NOSC in each of the five reserve regions. Leadership and policy oversight are provided by the Director of Psychological Health for the Navy Reserve assigned to the BUMED Deployment Health office. He or she is also responsible for coordinating with the Navy Reserve Forces Command and the Office of Chief of Naval Reserve; coordinating the development of the Navy Reserve Psychological Health strategic plan; monitoring the availability, accessibility, quality, and effectiveness of mental health services available to Navy reservists and their families; and developing the OSC education and training opportunities for reservists.

Table B.3—Continued

Feature	Description
Implementation history	In December 2007, the Navy Bureau of Medicine secured funding (PH and TBI funding to the Navy by Pub. L. 110-28) for a psychological health program to support naval reserves and returning warriors. Funding was awarded in 2008 to begin the Psychological Health Outreach program. Between January and May 2009, the psychological health outreach coordinators made 77 NOSC visits and provided education and training to more than 7,200 Reserve Corps members and NOSC staff; 471 clients received clinical assessment referral and follow-up. BUMED is planning to expand the program to the Marine Corps Reserves. A contract for the program expansion was approved in July 2009. Program expansion will include an additional 30 outreach coordinators and team members for the Marine Corps, who will work hand-in-hand with existing naval program staff.
Initiative costs or resource requirements	There are two full-time psychological health outreach coordinators and a psychological health team of five (with at least two licensed social workers) at each of six Reserve Command Components that provide all the program activities. Funding for the program was estimated to be approximately $2.99 million per year. In addition, NOSC dedicates time for initial assessments of reservists and for periodic psychological health education and training on OSC.
Evaluation design and outcomes	Annual reporting is required of this grant-funded effort. To monitor program implementation and success, program staff track and report annually the number of reservists contacted through outreach, the number served as clients, and the number of cases closed.
IOM category	Selective (mental health clinical and psychological assessments) Universal (psychological health education)
Published information	None available
Managing office	BUMED Deployment Health office http://www.med.navy.mil/bumed/Pages/default.aspx

NOTE: PH = psychological health.

Table B.4
Command-Level Suicide-Prevention Program and Suicide-Prevention Coordinator

Feature	Description
Brief description	Commands are asked to develop a written crisis response plan outlining emergency contacts, phone guidance, and basic safety precautions to assist a sailor in distress. An SPC is appointed for each command to ensure that the required program components are in place. SPCs receive training on suicide prevention and the requirements for a command suicide-prevention program (training, outreach, and response plan).
Target outcomes	- All commands develop standard operating procedures for preventing and responding to suicide risk. - All commands work systematically to prevent suicide attempts and completions.
Target population	All active-duty sailors

Table B.4—Continued

Feature	Description
Setting and scope of initiative	The command-level suicide-prevention program is delivered at each command in a variety of settings, including, but not limited to, life skills, health promotions, and GMT.
Implementation history	A checklist is posted on the Navy's website to help guide commands and SPCs in the development and implementation of the command-level suicide-prevention program. The checklist recommends that the following ten components be in place: - an appropriate annual suicide-prevention training - suicide prevention as part of the life skills and health-promotion training - messages of concern sent by the senior leadership team to provide current information and guidance to all personnel on suicide prevention - a written crisis response plan outlining emergency procedures for helping a sailor in distress - local support resource contact information (e.g., chaplain) - personnel and supervisors with ready access to information about how to get help with personal problems (e.g., wallet card information) - procedures to facilitate access to services (e.g., time for appointments) - supervisors active in identifying personnel potentially in need of support (e.g., relationship problems) - a safety plan for helping distressed sailors until mental health services are available (e.g., removal of hazards) - a coordinated follow-up plan for personnel following mental health evaluation or use of other support services. At the time of this writing, most commands had an SPC but had not been able to put in place the above components.
Initiative costs or resource requirements	Not available, as most commands are still developing their prevention programs
Evaluation design and outcomes	None available
IOM category	Universal (training and leadership messages) Selective (standard procedures for dealing with a suicidal crisis)
Published information	The command and leaders' tool box, which contains a leaders' guide, suicide-prevention program checklist, relevant instructions, and poster downloads is available on the NAVPERS website: http://www.npc.navy.mil/CommandSupport/SuicidePrevention/CommandLeaders/
Managing office	Personal Readiness and Community Support Branch http://www.suicide.navy.mil

NOTE: NAVPERS = Navy Personnel Command.

Table B.5
Operational Stress Control

Feature	Description
Brief description	The OSC program provides training and practical decisionmaking tools for sailors, leaders, and families to help them identify stress responses, mitigate problematic stress, and build resilience.
Target outcomes	- Address stress problems for sailors and their families early, when shipmates and leaders can mitigate the effects of stress. - Facilitate access to professional counseling or treatment needed by the sailor or family member (or both) and return the sailor back to the command. - Build resiliency among all sailors and their families, as well as commands, to ensure that they are mission-ready.
Target population	Active-duty sailors and their families
Setting and scope of initiative	The OSC program is based on a stress continuum model that is taught in a variety of settings. Three modules currently teach the stress continuum model: - OSC Awareness Training delivered to sailors during their Battlestation training in boot camp, as part of pre- and postdeployment training, and through a variety of additional ad hoc training opportunities - Navy Family Program, which provides communications, outreach, resource referral, information, and advocacy to and for command families through an appointed ombudsman - Care Giver OCS Training.
Implementation history	OSC became an official naval program in November 2008. However, training and education efforts related to OSC had been ongoing since 2007. At the time of this writing, the OSC Awareness Training had been provided to more than 70,000 sailors through the FFSC programs, the Reserve Psychological Outreach program, mobilization processing sites, Warrior Transition program in Kuwait, RWWs, MTF programs, and chaplains' professional development training courses. NETC uses a variety of media for this ongoing training. The Navy Family Program began integrating OSC into its operations in November 2009. The Care Giver OCS Training also began in November 2009.
Initiative costs or resource requirements	Not available, as the OSC initiative is still in development
Evaluation design and outcomes	None available
IOM category	Universal Selective (Care Giver OSC Training)
Published information	None available
Managing office	Operational Stress Control, Chief of Navy Personnel, U.S. Navy http://www.navy.mil/cnp/index.asp

Table B.6
Personal Readiness Summit and Fleet Suicide-Prevention Conference and Summit

Feature	Description
Brief description	Summits are in-person, half-day (minimum) training programs focused on bringing information to behavioral health professionals, chaplains, first responders, and command-appointed SPCs. Personal Readiness Summits focus broadly on OSC, alcohol- and drug-abuse prevention, physical readiness, and sexual-assault prevention and are supplemented by breakout sessions on these specific topic areas. The Fleet Suicide Prevention Conferences and Summits provide more-focused training on suicide prevention and opportunities for attendees to hear from invited speakers and network with support personnel and first responders.
Target outcomes	- Improve leader, command SPC, and installation first-responder awareness of emerging and best practices related to personal and fleet readiness. - Build on the skills learned at the annual suicide-prevention training.
Target population	Active-duty sailors in chaplaincy, behavioral health, first responder, and command-appointed SPC positions
Setting and scope of initiative	Summits and conferences are organized at areas of fleet concentration by a small group of two to three trainers.
Implementation history	This initiative began officially in 2008. As the alcohol-abuse prevention unit evolved into a more broadly focused personnel and family readiness division, the training supported by this unit also broadened. Summits were conducted in FY 2009 in Pearl Harbor (Hawaii), Norfolk (Va.), Jacksonville (Fla.), Mayport (Fla.), Kitsap (Wash.), Atsugi (Japan), Yokosuka (Japan), San Diego (Calif.), Port Hueneme (Calif.), Gulfport (Miss.), Groton (Conn.), Sigonella (Sicily), and Naples (Italy).
Initiative costs or resource requirements	Summit attendees are required to commit a half-day or more to attend. In addition, personnel resources support the organization and delivery of summit and conference material, as well as conference speakers from within and outside the Navy.
Evaluation design and outcomes	Trainers administer pre- and posttest evaluation questionnaires to assess whether trainees have learned the summit content and to evaluate how well the content was delivered. These questionnaires are required to ask about trainees' confidence level in helping a sailor in distress. However, they are not standardized across training modules and, at the time of this writing, had not yet been evaluated.
IOM category	Selective
Published information	None available
Managing office	Personal Readiness and Community Support Branch http://www.suicide.navy.mil

Table B.7
First-Responder Seminar

Feature	Description
Brief description	The first-responder seminar is a pilot project to provide installation first responders and support personnel (e.g., medical, security, chaplains, FFSC, dispatch, EMS) an opportunity to review deescalation and safety procedures when responding to a sailor in crisis. The seminar provides discussion of case examples and outlines how the various responder roles should work together.
Target outcomes	Improve first responders' knowledge of deescalation and safety considerations during a crisis.
Target population	Active-duty naval-installation first responders and support personnel
Setting and scope of initiative	The seminars were piloted for the first time by two to three trainers during the personal readiness summits in FY 2009.
Implementation history	The first-responder seminars were developed to fill a gap in the Navy's overall training program identified during a case review of an individual's death while in security custody. At the time of this writing, the curriculum was still in development.
Initiative costs or resource requirements	Not available, as the seminar series curriculum is still in final development
Evaluation design and outcomes	None available
IOM category	Selective
Published information	None available
Managing office	Personal Readiness and Community Support Branch http://www.suicide.navy.mil Commander Navy Installations Command http://www.cnic.navy.mil/CNIC_HQ_Site/index.htm

NOTE: EMS = emergency medical services.

Table B.8
Returning Warriors Workshops

Feature	Description
Brief description	The RWWs are weekend retreats for reservists who have recently returned from deployment as individual augmentees and their spouses. The workshops are designed to honor returning sailors and help ameliorate feelings of stress, isolation, and other psychological and physical injuries, especially PTSD and TBI. The workshops are delivered through group presentations, small group breakout sessions, informational sessions, and one-on-one counseling in a conference-style setting away from the military environment. Workshop facilitators are senior officers and enlisted personnel in the medical and social-work fields, as well as chaplains trained to help participants through potentially sensitive and emotional discussions.
Target outcomes	- Engage reservists and families in facilitated discussion to reduce feelings of stress and isolation. - Connect reservists to needed resources through contact with clinical outreach staff. - Assist reservists and families in identifying any immediate and potential psychological or physical health issues.
Target population	Qualifying participants include reservists who served as an individual augmentee since the September 11 terrorist attack and their spouses, or, if unmarried, significant others or close family members.
Setting and scope of initiative	Reservists enter the program through self-referral or referral by unit CO or spouse. Psychological health outreach coordinators inform reservists and COs about the program through briefings, visits, and letters to NOSC. Workshops are held away from the military environment in hotels and other conference venues across the country.
Implementation history	The RWW program is funded through the PH and TBI funding allocated to the Navy through Pub. L. 110-28. The workshops began in 2007, and, by May 2009, a total of 22 RWWs had been held, attended by 2,358 reservists and family members. Before grant funding ends in 2010, the BUMED Deployment Health Office plans to hold 27 additional workshops. At the time of this writing, the RWW was not a permanent program, and BUMED was providing additional funding to support the program while staff identify a more permanent home for the program.
Initiative costs or resource requirements	Initiative costs include (1) participating reservists' overnight stay in a high-quality hotel and accrediting them a weekend of drill pay; (2) guest-speaker travel and accommodations; (3) facilitators' training, time, travel, and accommodations; and (3) event-planning staff and venue costs. For 20 workshops, the estimated cost was $2.8 million.
Evaluation design and outcomes	Annual reporting was required of this grant-funded effort. To monitor program implementation and success, program staff annually tracked and reported on the number of reservists and family members who attended the RWW. Workshop evaluations from reservist participants were used to measure participant satisfaction, while results from after-action reports reflected staff perceptions of successes and challenges.
IOM category	Selective
Published information	None available
Managing office	BUMED Deployment Health Office http://www.med.navy.mil/bumed/Pages/default.aspx

Table B.9
Front-Line Supervisor Training

Feature	Description
Brief description	Front-line supervisor training is an interactive, half-day workshop designed for front-line leaders (i.e., NCOs and lieutenants) to recognize and respond to sailors in distress. The training includes case examples and role-play and is intended to expand on annual awareness training.
Target outcomes	- Improve sailors' ability to recognize and respond to other sailors in distress. - Reduce suicide attempts and suicides.
Target population	Active-duty sailors
Setting and scope of initiative	Training is delivered to the front-line supervisors in each command by their designated SPC.
Implementation history	The front-line supervisor training was developed jointly in the DoD SPARRC and has been implemented in the Navy via the Behavioral Health Program in the Personal Readiness and Community Support Branch. A train-the-trainer model has been used to facilitate rollout of this initiative since 2008. Train-the-trainer sessions have been provided by behavioral health staff at 16 locations throughout the world, and additional train-the-trainer sessions have been offered by fleet- and force-level SPCs. This training is just beginning to reach the fleet, and there are plans to continue expanding its reach by offering additional train-the-trainer sessions in 2010.
Initiative costs or resource requirements	One staff member per command is trained to deliver this module. This requires four hours of time from both the behavioral health staff member trainer and SPC trainee. In addition, command needs to provide a half-day for SPCs to deliver the training to all front-line supervisors.
Evaluation design and outcomes	Pre- and posttraining questionnaire
IOM category	Universal
Published information	None available
Managing office	Personal Readiness and Community Support Branch http://www.suicide.navy.mil

Air Force Suicide-Prevention Initiatives

Table C.1
Air Force Suicide Prevention Program

Feature	Description
Brief description	The AFSPP is a comprehensive, community-based approach for preventing suicide. It focuses on decreasing risk factors for suicide and enhancing protective factors, including promoting mental health treatment for those in need.
Target outcomes	- Promote awareness of risk factors related to suicide. - Educate the Air Force community regarding available mental health services. - Reduce stigma related to help-seeking behavior.
Target population	The entire Air Force community (including civilian employees)
Setting and scope of initiative	The 11 initiatives that comprise the AFSPP aim to strengthen social support, promote effective coping skills, and encourage help-seeking behavior.
Implementation history	The AFSPP was developed in 1996. An official evaluation was published in a peer-reviewed medical journal in 2003 (Knox et al., 2003). It is classified as a promising practice in the SPRC's Registry of Evidence-Based Suicide Prevention Programs and is listed on SAMHSA's NREPP.
Initiative costs or resource requirements	Unknown
Evaluation design and outcomes	Knox et al. (2003) found a 33% reduction in suicides after the program was implemented in the Air Force. An AFSPP checklist was developed to ensure that each installation is completing each of the 11 initiatives of the program. The checklist for each installation is signed by the IDS chair, the CAIB executive director, and the CAIB chair.
IOM category	Universal
Published information	- Knox et al. (2003) - AFPAM 44-160
Managing office	Air Force Medical Operations Agency 1780 Air Force Pentagon Washington DC 20330-1780 http://www.airforcemedicine.afms.mil ATTN: Air Force SPPM (as of this writing, Lt. Col. Michael Kindt, Michael.Kindt@LACKLAND.AF.MIL)

Table C.2
Assessing and Managing Suicide Risk Training for Mental Health Clinical Staff

Feature	Description
Brief description	Assessing and Managing Suicide Risk is a one-day workshop for mental health clinical staff that focuses on competencies that are core to assessing and managing suicide risk. The training was developed collaboratively by the AAS and the SPRC. The course encourages discussion and reflection on the complex ethical issues that must be considered when providing care to suicidal clients. Additionally, the course introduces the principles of CASE, a method for identifying suicidal ideation. Training is delivered through lecture, video demonstrations, and exercises. A 110-page participant manual is also handed out to participants.
Target outcomes	Mental health clinical staff will have the core competencies needed to assess and manage suicide risk.
Target population	Mental health providers that service active-duty airmen (Air Force)
Setting and scope of initiative	The training was offered by trainers at the SPRC.
Implementation history	Training was offered to mental health providers over a one-year period in 2007 with an informal plan to sustain training.
Initiative costs or resource requirements	Unknown
Evaluation design and outcomes	None available
IOM category	Selective
Published information	Information on the training is available on the SPRC website (http://www.sprc.org/traininginstitute/amsr/clincomp.asp).
Managing office	Air Force Medical Operations Agency 1780 Air Force Pentagon Washington DC 20330-1780 http://www.airforcemedicine.afms.mil

NOTE: CASE = Chronological Assessment of Suicide Events.

Table C.3
Landing Gear

Feature	Description
Brief description	The Landing Gear program serves as a standardized preexposure preparation training program for deploying airmen, as well as the mental health component of reintegration education for returning airmen. During the predeployment training, airmen learn about deployment stress, the deployed environment, typical reactions to combat and other deployment-related experiences, reintegration and reunion, prevention, and accessing help. The postdeployment training focuses on the same topics as the predeployment training but emphasizes typical reactions, reintegration and reunion and accessing help. Mental health personnel or qualified IDS members typically deliver the briefing. The training sessions are provided as a freestanding class or in conjunction with other briefings provided by the Airman and Family Readiness Center and chaplaincy.
Target outcomes	Landing Gear serves as a bridge to care services. It is designed to better support airmen suffering from traumatic stress symptoms and connect them with helping resources.
Target population	Airmen who will deploy or have deployed and are experiencing deployment-related trauma
Setting and scope of initiative	Sessions are held pre- and postdeployment and may be recurring as needed for larger groups scheduled to deploy or redeploy, or impromptu for individuals or groups with short-notice deployments or unanticipated returns.
Implementation history	Released in 2008
Initiative costs or resource requirements	Unknown
Evaluation design and outcomes	None available
IOM category	Indicated
Published information	Information on the program is available on the AFSPP website (http://afspp.afms.mil).
Managing office	Air Force Office of the Surgeon General 1780 Air Force Pentagon Washington DC 20330-1780 http://www.sg.af.mil ATTN: As of 2008, Lt. Col. Steven Pflanz (Steven.Pflanz@Pentagon.af.mil)

Marine Corps Suicide-Prevention Initiatives

Table D.1
Annual Suicide-Prevention Awareness Training

Feature	Description
Brief description	MCO 1700.24B requires annual suicide-prevention awareness training for all marines. The training is intended to provide all marines with knowledge and action strategies needed to understand and recognize suicidal risk among other marines. The following topics are covered during the training: definition of *suicide* and *suicide attempt*, prevalence of suicide completion in the Marine Corps, risk factors and warning signs for suicide, first-responder process, and relevant suicide resources.
Target outcomes	- All marines can define *suicide* and related terms. - All marines can identify risk factors and warning signs for suicide. - All marines know how to be a first responder.
Target population	Active-duty and reserve marines
Setting and scope of initiative	All marines are required by MCO 1700.24B to receive suicide awareness training annually.
Implementation history	The Marine Corps has required annual awareness training in suicide prevention since 1997. The Marine Corps Training and Education Command works with the MCSPP office in Manpower and Reserve Affairs to develop training materials. The training sessions are supplemented with information on local procedures and resources. Across the Marine Corps, local commands decide where and when to implement the training and have numerous choices of training format. MCSPP provides resources, such as videos, PowerPoint presentations, and distance learning courses. To allow commands to tailor the training for their specific populations, the Marine Corps does not require the use of a specific standardized tool.
Initiative costs or resource requirements	HQMC staff time is devoted to periodically updating available resources, while local commands provide time for integrating local procedures and resources into the training. In addition, all marines must be given time to attend the training.
Evaluation design and outcomes	None available
IOM category	Universal
Published information	None available
Managing office	Headquarters, Marine Corps Marine Corps Suicide Prevention Program (MCSPP) http://www.usmc-mccs.org/suicideprevent/

Table D.2
Public Information Materials on Suicide

Feature	Description
Brief description	The Marine Corps produced a website, posters, brochures, videos, and a play to offer information on the signs and symptoms of suicide and available resources and to reduce the stigma of getting help.
Target outcomes	Educate all marines on the signs and symptoms of suicide and available resources.

Table D.2—Continued

Feature	Description
Target population	All active-duty marines
Setting and scope of initiative	The communications are delivered through a variety of media, including these: - Website: The website contains a number of web-based resources to raise suicide awareness; links for online classes in which providers can earn continuing education units for suicide-related trainings; suicide-prevention briefing materials and resource guides for chaplains or medical and mental health providers; and links to suicide-prevention hotlines and Military OneSource. - Poster: The purpose of the poster is to raise awareness of suicide. It includes military and national statistics, as well as information about where marines in distress can seek assistance. The poster is available online, and copies of the poster are distributed to each installation for display in high-traffic areas, such as a gas station, commissary, or gym. - Brochure: A suicide-prevention brochure is available both online and at MCCS centers. - Informational videos: Videos that address the signs and symptoms of suicide are available. Informational videos are available for viewing online or on DVD by request. - Senior-leadership videos: All commanders were required to produce a short video with suicide prevention as part of the message. - Leaders Guide for Managing Marines in Distress (MCCS, undated [a]): a website and pocket guide with tools to help leaders address a range of problems (e.g., alcohol, relationships), including suicide - Play: All installations receive a copy of a play written and performed by marines and a 40-minute video performance of the play, which is a drama on suicide prevention.
Implementation history	The website was launched in 1998 and redesigned in 2007. The leaders' guide was first published in 2005. Pocket versions of the guide are available from Military OneSource. MARADMIN 134/09 required that, by March 15, 2009, every commanding office (i.e., colonels and generals) had to produce a suicide-prevention video (senior-leadership video) for its marines. The video was accompanied by a 2-hour required training on suicide prevention. In addition, a new video that contains personal accounts of suicide attempts and the family impact of suicide completions was finished in December 2009.
Initiative costs or resource requirements	Unknown
Evaluation design and outcomes	None available
IOM category	Universal
Published information	The suicide awareness and prevention website (http://www.usmc-mccs.org/suicideprevent/) contains links to the poster, brochure, and videos.
Managing office	Personal and Family Readiness Division of U.S. Marine Corps Manpower and Reserve Affairs http://www.usmc-mccs.org/suicideprevent http://www.usmc-mccs.org/leadersguide

Table D.3
Combat Operational Stress Control

Feature	Description
Brief description	The COSC program offers training to promote awareness of stress-related injuries and illness caused by combat or other operations, as well to teach marines and their families the skills needed to understand and combat stress. The COSC program also produces informational materials to support its training and education efforts. For example, the Combat Operational Stress Decision Flowchart (http://www.usmc-mccs.org/cosc/coscContMatrixMarines.cfm?sid=ml&smid=6&ssmid=1) is a tool that Marine leaders at all levels can use to assess the well-being of marines and their family members.
Target outcomes	- Maintain a ready fighting force. - Protect and restore the health of marines and their family members.
Target population	All active-duty and reserve marines
Setting and scope of initiative	Training and educational sessions are delivered at each installation and are integrated into Marine Corps schools, in addition to unit training throughout the deployment cycle. The COSC program also hosts an annual conference to present and critically examine COSC policies, programs, and practices specifically tailored to marines and their families.
Implementation history	The COSC program was formally established in 2006, and the stress continuum model provides the foundation for COSC programs and policies in the Marine Corps. The Marine Corps TECOM supports the COSC program by producing the workshops, videos, and other training materials needed.
Initiative costs or resource requirements	Unknown
Evaluation design and outcomes	None available
IOM category	Universal
Published information	The COSC program has a website (http://www.usmc-mccs.org/cosc/index.cfm?sid=ml&smid=1) linked to the Manpower and Reserve Affairs main page.
Managing office	U.S. Marine Corps Manpower and Reserve Affairs http://www.manpower.usmc.mil/

Table D.4
Suicide-Prevention Module for the Marine Corps Martial Arts Program

Feature	Description
Brief description	A 20-minute module on suicide awareness and prevention is integrated into Marine martial arts training. The module uses martial-arts metaphors to teach all marines about suicide prevention.
Target outcomes	All marines will be aware of the signs and symptoms of suicide and available resources.
Target population	All active-duty marines
Setting and scope of initiative	The module is implemented as part of a marine's regular, mandatory martial-arts training.
Implementation history	The MCMAP began in 2000. The Martial Arts Center of Excellence in Quantico developed the module in consultation with the Marine Corps SPPM. The suicide awareness and prevention module became a formal part of martial-arts training in 2008 but had been integrated into the training for several years prior.
Initiative costs or resource requirements	The module is integrated into an existing program infrastructure. Resources are needed to develop and update the module and train the existing instructors.
Evaluation design and outcomes	None available
IOM category	Universal
Published information	Program information can be found on the Martial Arts Center of Excellence website; however, information on the suicide awareness and prevention module is not published.
Managing office	Martial Arts Center of Excellence http://www.tecom.usmc.mil/mace/

Table D.5
Command-Level Suicide-Prevention Program, Suicide-Prevention Program Officers, and Installation-Level Suicide-Prevention Program Coordinators

Feature	Description
Brief description	Commands are asked to develop a suicide-prevention program that integrates and sustains awareness education, early identification and referral of at-risk personnel, treatment, and follow-up services. Annual suicide awareness training, postvention support, and suicide reporting using the DoDSER are also components of the program.
Target outcomes	- All commands develop a comprehensive program for preventing and responding to suicidal risk. - All commands implement their suicide-prevention program to systematically prevent suicide attempts and completions.
Target population	All active-duty marines
Setting and scope of initiative	The command-level suicide-prevention program is delivered at each command in a variety of settings, including, but not limited to, GMT.

Table D.5—Continued

Feature	Description
Implementation history	Marine Corps suicide-prevention programs have been required since 1997. Suicide-prevention measures are assessed through the Commanding General Inspection Program and by the Marine Corps Inspector General during every command inspection. A checklist is used to guide the assessment by HQMC: - an established suicide-prevention program that integrates and sustains awareness education, early identification and referral of at-risk personnel, treatment, and follow-up services - annual training in suicide awareness and prevention - trainers who demonstrate current knowledge about suicide prevention, use standardized training resources, and offer up-to-date information about local resources - evaluations by mental health professionals and appropriate follow-up for all personnel who make suicide gestures and attempts - reporting of all attempted suicides and suicide gestures by active-duty personnel (PCR) - a DoDSER on all cases of suicide deaths or undetermined deaths for which suicide has not been excluded - support to families and affected units after the suicide or suspected suicide of a marine. In November 2009, this checklist was in the process of being updated to reflect new reporting requirements in use by the DoDSER. MCSPP was planning to appoint an SPO for each command to ensure that all program components were in place. MCSPP also planned to appoint an SPC for each command to oversee SPOs and act as a resource for the Health Promotion Unit program offices. As of November 2009, no program officers or coordinators had been appointed.
Initiative costs or resource requirements	Not available
Evaluation design and outcomes	None available
IOM category	Universal (annual training) Selective (evaluation and follow-up by mental health professionals)
Published information	An AIRS detailed inspection checklist is available online at http://www.usmc-mccs.org/suicideprevent/.
Managing office	U.S. Marine Corps Manpower and Reserve Affairs http://www.manpower.usmc.mil/

Table D.6
Operational Stress Control and Readiness

Feature	Description
Brief description	The OSCAR program attempts to bridge the gap between behavioral health and military operations by embedding behavioral health professionals in infantry regiments. Behavioral health professionals act as OSC and COSC specialists who educate and are educated by their marines through repeated contact in the field and shared experiences before, during, and after deployment.
Target outcomes	- Reduce stigma associated with consulting with behavioral health professionals. - Increase awareness of OSC and COSC principles among marines. - Increase access to and provision of care needed to reduce long-term deployment-related stress problems.
Target population	All active-duty marines who are part of infantry divisions
Setting and scope of initiative	OSCAR behavioral health professionals are embedded in an active unit and serve the fellow marines in their unit, including when the unit is deployed.
Implementation history	The OSCAR program began in 1999 and was first implemented in the Second Marine Division at Camp Lejeune, North Carolina. In 2003, the Medical Officer of the Marine Corps championed the expansion of the OSCAR program to include all three marine infantry divisions. In November 2009, behavioral health professionals were being embedded into OSCAR teams on an ad hoc basis. The Marine Corps is currently evaluating the expansion of this program.
Initiative costs or resource requirements	Not available
Evaluation design and outcomes	None available
IOM category	Selective
Published information	A report on OSCAR has been published by Headquarters Marine Corps for Manpower and Reserve Affairs (Nash, 2006).
Managing office	Personal and Family Readiness Division of the Marine Corps Manpower and Reserve Affairs http://www.usmc-mccs.org/

Table D.7
Noncommissioned-Officer Suicide-Prevention Training Course

Feature	Description
Brief description	The NCO suicide-prevention course is a training course to educate NCOs about the impact of suicide and how to identify and intervene with a marine in distress. The course is built around 15 short videos that are supplemented with educational presentations and discussion of leadership responsibility, action, and commitment to suicide prevention.
Target outcomes	Every NCO understands how to prevent suicide and what his or her role is as a leader.
Target population	NCOs in the Marine Corps and Navy corpsmen who are part of USMC units
Setting and scope of initiative	The training is a half-day, peer-led program conducted by two sergeants at the unit level. All NCOs were trained using the course materials by October 30, 2009, and the course will continue to be a mandatory part of NCO training.
Implementation history	The curriculum was developed by NTEC in collaboration with MCSPP. In July and August 2009, eight regional master training teams traveled to Quantico to receive training by MCSPP and then went to regions to conduct the train-the-trainer courses with sergeants at each installation. Approximately 1,300 sergeant instructors were trained. Sergeant instructors were required to train all NCOs by the end of October and trained approximately 70,000 NCOs. The course will be sustained as a mandatory NCO training course.
Initiative costs or resource requirements	Unknown
Evaluation design and outcomes	The Uniformed Services University of the Health Sciences is currently evaluating the effectiveness of the NCO course. No results or reports were available in November 2009.
IOM category	Selective
Published information	Information on the training is available on the SPRC website (http://www.sprc.org/traininginstitute/amsr/clincomp.asp).
Managing office	Headquarters, Marine Corps Marine Corps Suicide Prevention Program (MCSPP) http://www.usmc-mccs.org/suicideprevent/ncotrng.cfm?sid=ml&smid=9

Table D.8
Entry-Level Training in Suicide Prevention

Feature	Description
Brief description	All entry-level marines (enlisted and officers) and their drill instructors are trained on suicide prevention. During boot camp, all enlisted marines are trained on the signs and symptoms of suicide and available resources. Training is delivered through two short courses and an interactive discussion led by a senior drill instructor. Officers receive training in suicide prevention through a brief module in officer candidate school and a short course in basic school. Suicide prevention is also discussed during two interactive discussions with a chaplain and an instructor (typically a lieutenant colonel). Drill instructors, responsible for boot-camp education, also receive specialized training on how to conduct an interactive discussion and are trained using the NCO suicide-prevention course curriculum. All entry-level training programs communicate the RACE model.
Target outcomes	- Upon entry into the Marine Corps, all marines are taught how to recognize and refer marines in distress. - All drill instructors supervising entry-level marines are trained in suicide prevention.
Target population	All active-duty marines
Setting and scope of initiative	Enlisted marines receive the entry-level training on suicide prevention during boot camp at the recruit training depots in Parris Island, South Carolina, or San Diego, California. Drill instructors receive training through the Marine Corps during their ten-week training course, also located at the training depot centers. Officers receive training during officer candidate school and basic school in Quantico, Virginia.
Implementation history	In October 2009, the enlisted entry-level training curriculum and the drill-instructor training curriculum were updated to expand focus on suicide prevention. Changes to the enlisted training included (1) separating suicide prevention into a stand-alone 30-minute module given at the end of boot camp (this occurs instead of the Warrior Preservation brief, in which the senior drill instructor informed Marines about potential risks of which to be aware during the week of leave that occurs after boot camp; (2) making the senior drill instructor responsible for the suicide-prevention briefing, rather than relying on the chaplain to conduct the briefing; and (3) adding some video clips from the NCO suicide-prevention course. Drill-instructor training was updated to include the NCO suicide-prevention course. At the time of this writing, TECOM was in the process of revising the officer training course.
Initiative costs or resource requirements	Unknown
Evaluation design and outcomes	None available
IOM category	Universal
Published information	None available
Managing office	U.S. Marine Corps Training and Education Command http://www.tecom.usmc.mil

NOTE: RACE = Recognize changes in your marine; ask your marine directly whether he or she is thinking about killing him- or herself; care for your marine by calmly controlling the situation, listening without judgment, and removing any means that the marine could use to inflict self-injury; and escort your marine to the chain of command, a chaplain, mental health professional, or primary-care provider.

Table D.9
Assessing and Managing Suicide Risk Training for Mental Health Providers, Counselors, and Chaplains

Feature	Description
Brief description	The Assessing and Managing Suicide Risk program is a one-day workshop for behavioral health professionals and chaplains that teaches how to assess and manage suicide risk. The training was developed collaboratively by the AAS and the SPRC, both civilian organizations. The course encourages discussion and reflection on the complex ethical issues that must be considered when providing care to suicidal individuals. Additionally, the course introduces the principles of CASE, a method for recognizing suicidal ideation. Training is delivered through lecture, video demonstrations, and exercises. A 110-page participant manual is also handed out to participants.
Target outcomes	Behavioral health professionals and chaplains will have the core competencies needed to assess and manage suicide risk.
Target population	Behavioral health professionals and chaplains who service active-duty marines
Setting and scope of initiative	The training is delivered on installations by a certified behavioral health officer.
Implementation history	A single behavioral health officer was certified in this training module and, during the 2008 calendar year, traveled to each Marine Corps installation to offer the training to mental health providers, chaplains, and counselors. At the time of this writing, there was no strategy in place to sustain the training.
Initiative costs or resource requirements	Unknown
Evaluation design and outcomes	None available
IOM category	Selective
Published information	Information on the training is available on the SPRC website.
Managing office	U.S. Marine Corps Manpower and Reserve Affairs http://www.manpower.usmc.mil/ http://www.usmc-mccs.org/suicideprevent/

Table D.10
Are You Listening?

Feature	Description
Brief description	This prevention program targets civilian staff affiliated with MCCS MWR facilities and teaches them to recognize and report marines in distress (suicide and alcohol problems). Staff include individuals who work at fitness (gym), shopping (military exchanges), and recreation facilities (golf courses, campgrounds, pools), as well as other service positions (e.g., car washes, gas stations, video stores). Staff attend a two-day training to help them understand - the current prevalence of risk behaviors reported in the Marine Corps annual health assessment (e.g., sexual assault, domestic violence, child abuse, and suicide) - the Marine Corps's current approach to prevention - the installation resources (financial assistance, mental health, medical, fitness, relocation, career transition, substance abuse, relationship) - how to apply active listening and communication skills to help intervene with a marine in distress. During the second day of training, participants design a sustainment plan to describe how they will continue to use the active listening techniques they developed during training. Most of the information for the training is excerpted from the Marine Corps "Leaders Guide for Managing Marines in Distress" (MCCS, undated [a]).
Target outcomes	Staff recognize and report marines in distress.
Target population	Staff affiliated with MCCS MWR facilities
Setting and scope of initiative	This program is delivered on Marine Corps installations. Staff are expected to implement the lessons learned during work.
Implementation history	The first pilot test of the training was conducted in 2007, and the training has been slowly rolling out to installations. Currently, the trainers are centralized at HQMC.
Initiative costs or resource requirements	Unknown
Evaluation design and outcomes	None available
IOM category	Universal
Published information	None available
Managing office	U.S. Marine Corps Manpower and Reserve Affairs http://www.manpower.usmc.mil/

Table D.11
Front-Line Supervisor Training

Feature	Description
Brief description	The front-line supervisor training is a voluntary, interactive half-day workshop designed to assist front-line leaders (i.e., NCOs) to recognize and respond to marines in distress. The training includes case examples and role-play and is intended to expand on annual awareness training.
Target outcomes	- Improve marines' ability to recognize and respond to other marines in distress. - Reduce suicides and suicide attempts.
Target population	NCO marines and others in front-line leadership positions
Setting and scope of initiative	Training is delivered to front-line supervisors either by a trained civilian instructor on each installation or by NCOs who have completed a train-the-trainer course at the installation.
Implementation history	The front-line supervisor training was developed jointly in the DoD SPARRC. Marine Corps Semper Fit health-promotion personnel are in charge of conducting training sessions as needed at all Marine Corps installations. These instructors conduct both train-the-trainer courses and direct training as required at the installation level. All installation Semper Fit trainers were trained and certified at the annual Military Suicide Prevention Conference in April 2008.
Initiative costs or resource requirements	Train-the-trainer courses require one day, and the front-line supervisor training course requires a half-day commitment.
Evaluation design and outcomes	None available
IOM category	Universal
Published information	None available
Managing office	Headquarters, Marine Corps Marine Corps Suicide Prevention Program (MCSPP) http://www.usmc-mccs.org/suicideprevent/

References

AFI 41-210—see U.S. Department of the Air Force (2006b [2010]).

AFI 44-109—*see* U.S. Department of the Air Force (2000).

AFI 44-153—*see* U.S. Department of the Air Force (2006c).

AFI 44-154—*see* U.S. Department of the Air Force (2003).

AFI 90-501—*see* U.S. Department of the Air Force (2006d).

AFMOA—*see* Air Force Medical Operations Agency.

AFPAM 44-160—*see* U.S. Department of the Air Force (2001).

Air Force Medical Operations Agency, Population Health Support Division, *Air Force Guide for Managing Suicidal Behavior: Strategies, Resources, and Tools,* undated. As of March 5, 2010: http://afspp.afms.mil/idc/groups/public/documents/afms/ctb_016017.pdf

Air Force Medical Service, undated web page. As of April 8, 2010: http://afspp.afms.mil/idc/groups/public/documents/webcontent/knowledgejunction.hcst? functionalarea=AFSuicidePreventionPrgm&doctype=folderlist&folderName=Memos&incbanner=0

Air Force Surgeon General, undated home page. As of March 16, 2010: http://www.sg.af.mil/

Allard, R., M. Marshall, and M. C. Plante, "Intensive Follow-Up Does Not Decrease the Risk of Repeat Suicide Attempts," *Suicide and Life-Threatening Behavior,* Vol. 22, No. 3, Fall 1992, pp. 303–314.

AMEDD—*see* U.S. Army Medical Department.

Anthony, James C., and M. L. Van Etten, "Epidemiology and Its Rubrics," in Alan S. Bellack, Michel Hersen, and C. Eugene Walker, eds., *Comprehensive Clinical Psychology,* Vol. 1: *Foundations,* New York: Pergamon, 1998, pp. 355–390.

Aoun, Samar, "Deliberate Self-Harm in Rural Western Australia: Results of an Intervention Study," *Australian and New Zealand Journal of Mental Health Nursing,* Vol. 8, No. 2, June 1999, pp. 65–73.

APHC—*see* U.S. Army Public Health Command (Provisional).

AR 600-24—*see* Headquarters Department of the Army (2009a).

AR 600-63—*see* Headquarters Department of the Army (2007 [2009]).

AR 600-85—*see* Headquarters Department of the Army (2009a).

"Army Will Investigate Recruiters' Suicides," *New York Times*, November 8, 2008, p. A32. As of March 5, 2010:
http://www.nytimes.com/2008/11/09/us/09recruiters.html

Aseltine, Robert H. Jr., Amy James, Elizabeth A. Schilling, and Jaime Glanovsky, "Evaluating the SOS Suicide Prevention Program: A Replication and Extension," *BioMed Central Public Health*, Vol. 7, July 18, 2007, p. 161. As of March 5, 2010:
http://www.biomedcentral.com/1471-2458/7/161

AskClyde, *Evaluation of Applied Suicide Intervention Skills Training (ASIST): West Dunbartonshire*, June 2007.

Barry, Sheila, "Pastoral Counseling in the Military," in Robert J. Wicks, Richard D. Parsons, and Donald Capps, eds., *Clinical Handbook of Pastoral Counseling*, Vol. 3, New York: Paulist Press, 2003, pp. 1–16.

Beautrais, A. L., P. R. Joyce, R. T. Mulder, D. M. Fergusson, B. J. Deavoll, and S. K. Nightingale, "Prevalence and Comorbidity of Mental Disorders in Persons Making Serious Suicide Attempts: A Case-Control Study," *American Journal of Psychiatry*, Vol. 153, August 1996, pp. 1009–1014.

Beck, Aaron T., and Robert A. Steer, *BHS, Beck Hopelessness Scale: Manual*, San Antonio, Texas: Psychological Corp., 1988.

Berman, A. L., "Fictional Depiction of Suicide in Television Films and Imitation Effects," *American Journal of Psychiatry*, Vol. 145, August 1988, pp. 982–986.

Birckmayer, J., and D. Hemenway, "Minimum-Age Drinking Laws and Youth Suicide, 1970–1990," *American Journal of Public Health*, Vol. 89, No. 9, September 1999, pp. 1365–1368.

Birkhead, G. S., V. G. Galvin, P. J. Meehan, P. W. O'Carroll, and J. A. Mercy, "The Emergency Department in Surveillance of Attempted Suicide: Findings and Methodologic Considerations," *Public Health Reports*, Vol. 108, No. 3, May–June 1993, pp. 323–331.

Blue Ribbon Work Group on Suicide Prevention in the Veteran Population, *Report to James B. Peake, MD, Secretary of Veterans Affairs*, Washington, D.C.: Department of Veterans Affairs, 2008.

Brady Campaign to Prevent Gun Violence, "State Gun Laws," undated web page. As of November 20, 2009:
http://www.bradycampaign.org/stategunlaws

Bray, Robert M., and Laurel L. Hourani, "Substance Use Trends Among Active Duty Military Personnel: Findings from the United States Department of Defense Health Related Behavior Surveys, 1980–2005," *Addiction*, Vol. 102, No. 7, July 2007, pp. 1092–1101.

Bray, Robert M., Laurel L. Hourani, Kristine L. Rae Olmsted, Michael Witt, Janice M. Brown, Michael R. Pemberton, Mary Ellen Marsden, Bernadette Marriott, Scott Scheffler, and Russ Vandermaas-Peeler, *2005 Department of Defense Survey of Health Related Behaviors Among Active Duty Military Personnel*, Fort Belvoir, Va.: Defense Technical Information Center, 2006. As of March 5, 2010:
http://handle.dtic.mil/100.2/ADA465678

Bray, Robert M., Michael R. Pemberton, Laurel L. Hourani, Michael Witt, Kristine L. Rae Olmsted, Janice M. Brown, BeLinda Weimer, Marian E. Lane, Mary Ellen Marsden, Scott Scheffler, Russ Vandermaas-Peeler, Kimberly R. Aspinwall, Erin Anderson, Kathryn Spagnola, Kelly Close, Jennifer L. Gratton, Sara Calvin, and Michael Bradshaw, *2008 Department of Defense Survey of Health Related Behaviors Among Active Duty Military Personnel*, Washington, D.C.: U.S. Department of Defense, 2009. As of March 5, 2010:
http://www.tricare.mil/2008HealthBehaviors.pdf

Brent, David A., "Selective Serotonin Reuptake Inhibitors and Suicidality: A Guide for the Perplexed," *Canadian Journal of Psychiatry*, Vol. 54, No. 2, February 2009, pp. 72–74; discussion 75.

Brent, David A., M. Baugher, J. Bridge, T. Chen, and L. Chiappetta, "Age- and Sex-Related Risk Factors for Adolescent Suicide," *Journal of the American Academy of Child and Adolescent Psychiatry*, Vol. 38, No. 12, December 1999, pp. 1497–1505.

Brent, David A., and J. John Mann, "Family Genetic Studies, Suicide, and Suicidal Behavior," *American Journal of Medical Genetics Part C: Seminars in Medical Genetics*, Vol. 133C, No. 1, February 15, 2005, pp. 13–24.

Brown, Gregory K., Aaron T. Beck, R. A. Steer, and J. R. Grisham, "Risk Factors for Suicide in Psychiatric Outpatients: A 20-Year Prospective Study," *Journal of Consulting and Clinical Psychology*, Vol. 68, No. 3, 2000, pp. 371–377.

Brown, Gregory K., Thomas Ten Have, Gregg R. Henriques, Sharon X. Xie, Judd E. Hollander, and Aaron T. Beck, "Cognitive Therapy for the Prevention of Suicide Attempts: A Randomized Controlled Trial," *Journal of the American Medical Association*, Vol. 294, No. 5, August 3, 2005, pp. 563–570.

Brown, Lt. Gen. Richard E. III, Acting Assistant Vice Chief of Staff, U.S. Air Force, "Re-Energize Community Action Information Boards (CAIBs) and Integrated Delivery Systems (IDSs)," memorandum for vice commanders, headquarters Air Combat Command, Air Education and Training Command, Air Force Materiel Command, Air Force Space Command, Air Force Special Operations Command, Air Force Reserve Command, Air National Guard, Air Mobility Command, Pacific Air Forces, and U.S. Air Forces in Europe, and vice commander 11th Air Wing, June 22, 2004.

Bruce, Martha L., E. L. Brown, P. J. Raue, A. E. Mlodzianowski, B. S. Meyers, A. C. Leon, M. Heo, A. L. Byers, R. L. Greenberg, S. Rinder, W. Katt, and P. Nassisi, "A Randomized Trial of Depression Assessment Intervention in Home Health Care," *Journal of the American Geriatrics Society*, Vol. 55, No. 11, November 2007, pp. 1793–1800.

Bruce, Martha L., Thomas R. Ten Have, Charles F. Reynolds III, Ira I. Katz, Herbert C. Schulberg, Benoit H. Mulsant, Gregory K. Brown, Gail J. McAvay, Jane L. Pearson, and George S. Alexopoulos, "Reducing Suicidal Ideation and Depressive Symptoms in Depressed Older Primary Care Patients," *Journal of the American Medical Association*, Vol. 291, No. 9, March 3, 2004, pp. 1081–1091.

Bryan, Craig J., Luther E. Dhillon-Davis, and Kieran K. Dhillon-Davis, "Emotional Impact of a Video-Based Suicide Prevention Program on Suicidal Viewers and Suicide Survivors," *Suicide and Life-Threatening Behavior*, Vol. 39, No. 6, December 2009, pp. 623–632.

Bunch, J., "Recent Bereavement in Relation to Suicide," *Journal of Psychosomatic Research*, Vol. 16, No. 5, August 1972, pp. 361–366.

Bunch, J., B. Barraclough, B. Nelson, and P. Sainsbury, "Suicide Following Bereavement of Parents," *Social Psychiatry and Psychiatric Epidemiology*, Vol. 6, No. 4, December 1971, pp. 193–199.

Burnam, M. Audrey, Lisa S. Meredith, Todd C. Helmus, Rachel M. Burns, Robert A. Cox, Elizabeth D'Amico, Laurie T. Martin, Mary E. Vaiana, Kayla M. Williams, and Michael R. Yochelson, "Systems of Care: Challenges and Opportunities to Improve Access to High-Quality Care," in Terri Tanielian and Lisa H. Jaycox, eds., *Invisible Wounds of War: Psychological and Cognitive Injuries, Their Consequences, and Services to Assist Recovery*, Santa Monica, Calif.: RAND Corporation, MG-720-CCF, 2008, pp. 245–428. As of March 5, 2010: http://www.rand.org/pubs/monographs/MG720/

Carter, Gregory L., Kerrie Clover, Ian M. Whyte, Andrew H. Dawson, and Catherine D'Este, "Postcards from the EDge Project: Randomised Controlled Trial of an Intervention Using Postcards to Reduce Repetition of Hospital Treated Deliberate Self Poisoning," *BMJ*, Vol. 331, No. 7520, October 8, 2005, p. 805.

———, "Postcards from the EDge: 24-Month Outcomes of a Randomised Controlled Trial for Hospital-Treated Self-Poisoning," *British Journal of Psychiatry*, Vol. 191, December 2007, pp. 548–553.

Cartwright, Jim, "ACE," presentation, U.S. Department of Defense/Veterans Affairs Suicide Prevention Conference, San Antonio, Texas, January 15, 2009.

Cavanagh, J. T. O., A. J. Carson, M. Sharpe, and S. M. Lawrie, "Psychological Autopsy Studies of Suicide: A Systematic Review," *Psychological Medicine*, Vol. 33, No. 3, April 2003, pp. 395–405.

Cavanagh, J. T. O., D. G. C. Owens, and E. C. Johnstone, "Life Events in Suicide and Undetermined Death in South-East Scotland: A Case-Control Study Using the Method of Psychological Autopsy," *Social Psychiatry and Psychiatric Epidemiology*, Vol. 34, No. 12, December 1999, pp. 645–650.

CDC—*see* Centers for Disease Control and Prevention.

Cedereke, M., K. Monti, and A. Öjehagen, "Telephone Contact with Patients in the Year After a Suicide Attempt: Does It Affect Treatment Attendance and Outcome? A Randomised Controlled Study," *European Psychiatry*, Vol. 17, No. 2, April 2002, pp. 82–91.

Centers for Disease Control and Prevention, National Center for Injury Prevention and Control, "Data Sources for WISQARS™ Fatal," last reviewed September 7, 2006. As of November 17, 2009: http://www.cdc.gov/ncipc/wisqars/fatal/help/datasources.htm

———, "Welcome to WISQARS™," last updated March 4, 2010. As of November 17, 2009: http://www.cdc.gov/injury/wisqars/index.html

Chavez, B. R., "Navy Suicide Prevention Program Direction, Initiatives, and Resources," document provided to the authors, 2009a.

———, "Suicide Prevention Communication Strategy," briefing slides provided to the authors, 2009b.

Cherpitel, C. J., "Substance Use, Injury, and Risk-Taking Dispositions in the General Population," *Alcoholism: Clinical and Experimental Research*, Vol. 23, No. 1, January 1999, pp. 121–126.

Chiarelli, GEN Peter W., Vice Chief of Staff, U.S. Army, "Army Campaign Plan for Health Promotion, Risk Reduction and Suicide Prevention (ACPHP)," memorandum to principal officials of Headquarters, Department of the Army, April 16, 2009.

Chief of Naval Operations, Department of the Navy, Suicide Prevention, NAVADMIN 243/05, September 26, 2005. As of March 5, 2010: http://www.npc.navy.mil/NR/rdonlyres/CFCFD185-24DC-4CBA-B21F-50943C7E9AF7/0/NAV05243.txt

———, Combat and Operational Stress Control and Warrior Transition Program Implementation, NAVADMIN 182/07, July 23, 2007. As of March 5, 2010: http://www.npc.navy.mil/NR/rdonlyres/03FA150C-9F2B-427B-9DE9-7873F19ED123/0/NAV07182.txt

———, FY-09 General Military Training (GMT), NAVADMIN 033/09, January 26, 2009a. As of March 5, 2010: http://www.npc.navy.mil/NR/rdonlyres/DE3A7ADC-32C3-494E-9A05-8C94F429CBBE/0/NAV09033.txt

————, Suicide and Suicide Attempt Reporting, NAVADMIN 122/09, April 23, 2009b. As of March 5, 2010:
http://www.npc.navy.mil/NR/rdonlyres/64265B30-750D-4E3A-A8FF-9D95A3ECDB5F/0/NAV09122.txt

CHPPM—*see* U.S. Army Center for Health Promotion and Preventive Medicine.

Christensen, Helen, Kathleen M. Griffiths, and Anthony F. Jorm, "Delivering Interventions for Depression by Using the Internet: Randomised Controlled Trial," *British Medical Journal*, Vol. 328, No. 7434, January 31, 2004, p. 265.

Clark, David A., Aaron T. Beck, and Brad A. Alford, *Scientific Foundations of Cognitive Theory and Therapy of Depression*, New York: John Wiley, 1999.

CNIC—*see* Commander, Navy Installations Command.

CNO—*see* Chief of Naval Operations.

Coffey, C. Edward, "Building a System of Perfect Depression Care in Behavioral Health," *Joint Commission Journal on Quality and Patient Safety*, Vol. 33, No. 4, April 2007, pp. 193–199.

Colorado Trust, *Gatekeepers: Helping to Prevent Suicide in Colorado: An Evaluation Report on the Preventing Suicide in Colorado Initiative*, December 2007. As of March 16, 2010:
http://www.coloradotrust.org/attachments/0000/3095/COT_SuicidePrevInCOvF.pdf

Commandant of the Marine Corps, Department of Defense Suicide Event Report, Marine administrative message 147/08, February 28, 2008. As of March 5, 2010:
http://www.usmc.mil/news/messages/Pages/MESSAGES140.aspx

————, All Hands Suicide Prevention Training, Marine administrative message 134/09, February 2009a.

————, Twenty-First Executive Safety Board (ESB) Results, Marine administrative message 364/09, June 12, 2009b. As of March 8, 2010:
http://www.marines.mil/news/messages/Pages/MARADMIN0364-09.aspx

————, Noncommissioned Officer (NCO) Suicide Prevention Course Implementation Plan, Marine administrative message 404/09, July 2009c.

————, Modification to the Noncommissioned Officer (NCO) Suicide Prevention Course Implementation Plan, Marine administrative message 436/09, July 27, 2009d. As of March 5, 2010:
http://www.marines.mil/news/messages/Pages/MARADMIN0436-09.aspx

————, Program Evaluation Requirements ICO NCO Suicide Prevention Course, Marine administrative message 596/09, October 2009e. As of March 8, 2010:
http://www.marines.mil/news/messages/Pages/MARADMIN0596-09.aspx

Commander, Navy Installations Command, undated home page. As of March 16, 2010:
http://www.cnic.navy.mil/CNIC_HQ_Site/index.htm

Crosby, A. E., and L. Ortega, "Self-Directed Violence Surveillance: Uniform Definitions and Recommended Data Elements," paper presented at Suicidality and Risk of Suicidality: Definition, Drug Safety Concerns and a Necessary Target for Drug Development, Boston, Mass., March 23, 2009.

Cutler, David M., Edward L. Glaeser, and Karen E. Norberg, "Explaining the Rise in Youth Suicide," in Jonathan Gruber, ed., *Risky Behavior Among Youths: An Economic Analysis*, Chicago: University of Chicago Press, 2001, pp. 219–269.

DA PAM 600-24—*see* Headquarters Department of the Army (2009b).

DA PAM 600-70—*see* U.S. Army (1985).

Dahms, COL Jonathan, Office of the Chief of Public Affairs, "Army Campaign Plan for Health Promotion, Risk Reduction and Suicide Prevention," April 27, 2009. As of March 15, 2010: http://www.army.mil/-news/2009/04/27/ 20208-army-campaign-plan-for-health-promotion-risk-reduction-and-suicide-prevention/

DCoE—*see* Defense Centers of Excellence for Psychological Health and Traumatic Brain Injury.

De Leo, D., S. Burgis, J. M. Bertolote, A. J. Kerkhof, and U. Bille-Brahe, "Definitions of Suicidal Behavior: Lessons Learned from the WHO/EURO Multicentre Study," *Crisis*, Vol. 27, No. 1, 2006, pp. 4–15.

Defense Centers of Excellence for Psychological Health and Traumatic Brain Injury, "Real Warriors, Real Battles, Real Strength," undated web page. As of March 11, 2010: http://realwarriors.net/

———, "Suicide Prevention and Risk Reduction Committee (SPARRC): Suicide Overview," briefing slides provided to the authors, December 4, 2009.

Deputy Chief of Staff, Army G-1, "Suicide: Training," last updated November 4, 2009a. As of March 11, 2010: http://www.armyg1.army.mil/hR/suicide/training_sub.asp?sub_cat=20

———, "Suicide Prevention Training," last updated December 30, 2009b. As of March 11, 2010: http://www.armyg1.army.mil/hr/suicide/training.asp

———, "Suicide Prevention," last updated March 15, 2010. As of March 16, 2010: http://www.armyg1.army.mil/hr/suicide/

DoD—*see* U.S. Department of Defense.

Eaton, Danice K., Laura Kann, Steve Kinchen, James Ross, Joseph Hawkins, William A. Harris, Richard Lowry, Tim McManus, David Chyen, Shari Shanklin, Connie Lim, Jo Anne Grunbaum, and Howell Wechsler, "Youth Risk Behavior Surveillance: United States, 2005," *Morbidity and Mortality Weekly Report Surveillance Summaries*, Vol. 55, No. 5, June 9, 2006, pp. 1–108. As of March 8, 2010: http://www.cdc.gov/mmwr/preview/mmwrhtml/ss5505a1.htm

Eggert, Leona L., B. R. Randell, E. A. Thompson, and C. L. Johnson, *Washington State Youth Suicide Prevention Program: Report of Activities*, Seattle, Wash.: University of Washington, 2007.

Eggert, Leona L., E. A. Thompson, J. R. Herting, and L. J. Nicholas, "Reducing Suicide Potential Among High-Risk Youth: Tests of a School-Based Prevention Program," *Suicide and Life-Threatening Behavior*, Vol. 25, No. 2, Summer 1995, pp. 276–296.

Embrey, Ellen P., performing the duties of the Assistant Secretary of Defense (Health Affairs), "Report to Congress: Progress on Suicide Prevention," House report 110-652, June 2, 2009a.

———, "Reporting Guard and Reserve Component Suicides," memorandum for Gail H. McGinn, Deputy Under Secretary of Defense (Plans), July 2, 2009b.

Engel, Charles C., Thomas Oxman, Christopher Yamamoto, Darin Gould, Sheila Barry, Patrice Stewart, Kurt Kroenke, John W. Williams, and Allen J. Dietrich, "RESPECT-Mil: Feasibility of a Systems-Level Collaborative Care Approach to Depression and Post-Traumatic Stress Disorder in Military Primary Care," *Military Medicine*, Vol. 173, No. 10, October 2008, pp. 935–940.

EXORD 103-09—see Headquarters Department of the Army (2009b).

Farberow, N. L., H. K. Kang, and T. A. Bullman, "Combat Experience and Postservice Psychosocial Status as Predictors of Suicide in Vietnam Veterans," *Journal of Nervous and Mental Disease*, Vol. 178, No. 1, January 1990, pp. 32–37.

Fergusson, D. M., L. J. Woodward, and L. J. Horwood, "Risk Factors and Life Processes Associated with the Onset of Suicidal Behaviour During Adolescence and Early Adulthood," *Psychological Medicine*, Vol. 30, No. 1, January 2000, pp. 23–39.

Fisher, C. B., "Adolescent and Parent Perspectives on Ethical Issues in Youth Drug Use and Suicide Survey Research," *Ethics and Behavior*, Vol. 13, No. 4, 2003, pp. 303–332.

Fjeldsoe, Brianna S., Alison L. Marshall, and Yvette D. Miller, "Behavior Change Interventions Delivered by Mobile Telephone Short-Message Service," *American Journal of Preventive Medicine*, Vol. 36, No. 2, February 2009, pp. 165–173.

FM 22-51—*see* U.S. Department of the Army (1994).

FM 4-0—*see* Headquarters Department of the Army (2003).

Fu, Qiang, A. C. Heath, Kathleen K. Bucholz, Elliot C. Nelson, Anne L. Glowinski, J. Goldberg, M. J. Lyons, M. T. Tsuang, T. Jacob, M. R. True, and S. A. Eisen, "A Twin Study of Genetic and Environmental Influences on Suicidality in Men," *Psychological Medicine*, Vol. 32, 2002, pp. 11–24.

Gaskin, Thomas A., and CDR Edmond Feeks, "MARADMIN 112/07, the USMC Combat/ Operational Stress Control (COSC) Program, and the Post-Deployment Health Reassessment (PDHRA) Program," briefing, June 19, 2007. As of November 20, 2009: http://www.usmc-mccs.org/cosc/conf2007/documents/ 3C%20Combined%20Gaskin-Feeks%20COSC-PDHRA%20Brief%20070619.pdf

Gaynes, Bradley N., Suzanne L. West, Carol A. Ford, Paul Frame, Jonathan Klein, and Kathleen N. Lohr, "Screening for Suicide Risk in Adults: A Summary of the Evidence for the U.S. Preventive Services Task Force," *Annals of Internal Medicine*, Vol. 140, No. 10, May 18, 2004, pp. 822–835.

Gibb, Sheree J., Annette L. Beautrais, and David M. Fergusson, "Mortality and Further Suicidal Behaviour After an Index Suicide Attempt: A 10-Year Study," *Australian and New Zealand Journal of Psychiatry*, Vol. 39, No. 1–2, January 2005, pp. 95–100.

Glowinski, Anne L., Kathleen K. Bucholz, Elliot C. Nelson, Qiang Fu, Pamela A. F. Madden, Wendy Reich, and Andrew C. Heath, "Suicide Attempts in an Adolescent Female Twin Sample," *Journal of the American Academy of Child and Adolescent Psychiatry*, Vol. 40, No. 11, November 2001, pp. 1300–1307.

Goldsmith, Sara K., T. C. Pellman, A. M. Kleinman, and W. E. Bunney, eds., *Reducing Suicide: A National Imperative*, Washington, D.C.: National Academies Press, 2002.

Goode, Erica, "Suicide's Rising Toll: After Combat, Victims of an Inner War," *New York Times*, August 1, 2009, p. A1. As of March 8, 2010: http://www.nytimes.com/2009/08/02/us/02suicide.html

Gould, Madelyn S., "Teenage Suicide Clusters," *Journal of the American Medical Association*, Vol. 263, No. 15, April 18, 1990, p. 2051.

———, "Suicide and the Media," *Annals of the New York Academy of Sciences*, Vol. 932, April 2001, pp. 200–221; discussion pp. 221–204.

Gould, Madelyn S., John Kalafat, Jimmie Lou HarrisMunfakh, and Marjorie Kleinman, "An Evaluation of Crisis Hotline Outcomes, Part 2: Suicidal Callers," *Suicide and Life-Threatening Behavior*, Vol. 37, No. 3, June 2007, pp. 338–352.

Gould, Madelyn S., Frank A. Marrocco, Marjorie Kleinman, John Graham Thomas, Katherine Mostkoff, Jean Cote, and Mark Davies, "Evaluating Iatrogenic Risk of Youth Suicide Screening Programs: A Randomized Controlled Trial," *Journal of the American Medical Association*, Vol. 293, No. 13, April 6, 2005, pp. 1635–1643.

Gould, Madelyn S., D. Shaffer, and Marjorie Kleinman, "The Impact of Suicide in Television Movies: Replication and Commentary," *Suicide and Life-Threatening Behavior*, Vol. 18, No. 1, Spring 1988, pp. 90–99.

Gould, Madelyn S., Sylvan Wallenstein, and Marjorie Kleinman, "Time-Space Clustering of Teenage Suicide," *American Journal of Epidemiology*, Vol. 131, No. 1, January 1990, pp. 71–78.

Gould, Madelyn S., Sylvan Wallenstein, Marjorie H. Kleinman, P. O'Carroll, and J. Mercy, "Suicide Clusters: An Examination of Age-Specific Effects," *American Journal of Public Health*, Vol. 80, No. 2, February 1990, pp. 211–212.

Griesbach, Dawn, *The Use and Impact of Applied Suicide Intervention Skills Training (ASIST) in Scotland: An Evaluation*, Edinburg: Social Research, 2008.

Guo, B., and C. Harstall, *For Which Strategies of Suicide Prevention Is There Evidence of Effectiveness?* Copenhagen: World Health Organization Regional Office for Europe, Health Evidence Network report, July 2004. As of March 8, 2010:
http://www.euro.who.int/document/e83583.pdf

Hacker, K., J. Collins, L. Gross-Young, S. Almeida, and N. Burke, "Coping with Youth Suicide and Overdose: One Community's Efforts to Investigate, Intervene, and Prevent Suicide Contagion," *Crisis*, Vol. 29, No. 2, 2008, pp. 86–95.

Haley, R. W., "Point: Bias from the 'Healthy-Warrior Effect' and Unequal Follow-Up in Three Government Studies of Health Effects of the Gulf War," *American Journal of Epidemiology*, Vol. 148, No. 4, August 15, 1998, pp. 315–323.

Hall, Katherine, *Does Asking About Suicidal Ideation Increase the Likelihood of Suicide Attempts? A Critical Appraisal of the Literature*, Christchurch, N.Z.: New Zealand Health Technology Assessment, suicide prevention topic 7, 2002.

Hanzlick, R., "Coroner Training Needs: A Numeric and Geographic Analysis," *Journal of the American Medical Association*, Vol. 276, No. 21, December 4, 1996, pp. 1775–1778.

Harris, E. C., and B. Barraclough, "Suicide as an Outcome for Mental Disorders: A Meta-Analysis," *British Journal of Psychiatry*, Vol. 170, March 1997, pp. 205–228.

Hawton, Keith, "Sex and Suicide: Gender Differences in Suicidal Behaviour," *British Journal of Psychiatry*, Vol. 177, December 2000, pp. 484–485.

Hayward, L., S. R. Zubrick, and S. Silburn, "Blood Alcohol Levels in Suicide Cases," *Journal of Epidemiology and Community Health*, Vol. 46, No. 3, June 1992, pp. 256–260.

Headquarters Department of the Army, Sustainment, Army field manual 4-0, August 2003.

———, Leaders Guide for Suicide Prevention Planning, U.S. Army Training and Doctrine Command pamphlet 600-22, February 16, 2005. As of March 8, 2010:
http://www.tradoc.army.mil/tpubs/pams/p600-22.pdf

———, Army Health Promotion, Army regulation 600-63, May 7, 2007, rapid action revision issue date September 20, 2009. As of April 13, 2010:
http://www.army.mil/usapa/epubs/pdf/r600_63.pdf

———, The Army Substance Abuse Program, Army regulation 600-85, February 2, 2009a, rapid action revision issue date December 2, 2009. As of April 13, 2010:
http://www.army.mil/USAPA/epubs/pdf/r600_85.pdf

———, Army Suicide Prevention, executive order 103-09, February 10, 2009b.

———, Army Health Promotion, Army regulation 600-63, rapid action revision, issue date September 20, 2009c. As of April 8, 2010:
http://www.army.mil/usapa/epubs/pdf/r600_63.pdf

———, Health Promotion, Risk Reduction, and Suicide Prevention, Department of the Army pamphlet 600-24, December 17, 2009d. As of March 12, 2010:
http://www.army.mil/usapa/epubs/pdf/p600_24.pdf

Headquarters U.S. Marine Corps, Department of the Navy, "HQMC Organization Chart," undated.

———, Marine Corps Community Services Policy Manual, Marine Corps order P1700.27A, November 8, 1999a. As of March 8, 2010:
http://www.quantico.usmc.mil/download.aspx?Path=./Uploads/Files/FIN_MCO%20P1700.27A.pdf

———, Marine Corps Semper Fit Program Manual, Marine Corps order P1700.29, November 8, 1999b. As of March 8, 2010:
http://www.marines.mil/news/publications/Documents/MCO%20P1700.29.pdf

———, Marine Corps Personal Services Manual, Marine Corps order P1700.24B with change 1, December 27, 2001. As of March 8, 2010:
http://www.marines.mil/news/publications/Documents/
MCO%20P1700.24B%20W%20CH%201.pdf

———, Marine Corps Casualty Procedures Manual, Marine Corps order P3040.4E, February 27, 2003. As of March 8, 2010:
http://www.marines.mil/news/publications/Documents/MCO%20P3040.4E.pdf

———, Individual Training Standards (ITS) System for Marine Corps Common Skills (MCCS), Volume I, Marine Corps order 1510.89B, October 1, 2004. As of March 8, 2010:
http://www.usmc.mil/news/publications/Documents/MCO%201510.89B.pdf

Hedstrom, Peter, Ka-Yuet Liu, and Monica K. Nordvik, "Interaction Domains and Suicide: A Population-Based Panel Study of Suicides in Stockholm, 1991–1999," Social Forces, Vol. 87, No. 2, December 2008, pp. 713–740.

Hegerl, Ulrich, Lisa Wittenburg, Ella Arensman, Chantal Van Audenhove, James C. Coyne, David McDaid, Christina M. van der Feltz-Cornelis, Ricardo Gusmão, Mária Kopp, Margaret Maxwell, Ullrich Meise, Saska Roskar, Marco Sarchiapone, Armin Schmidtke, Airi Värnik, and Anke Bramesfeld, "Optimizing Suicide Prevention Programs and Their Implementation in Europe (OSPI Europe): An Evidence-Based Multi-Level Approach," BMC Public Health, Vol. 9, 2009, p. 428.

Henriksson, M. M., H. M. Aro, M. J. Marttunen, M. E. Heikkinen, E. T. Isometsä, K. I. Kuoppasalmi, and J. K. Lönnqvist, "Mental Disorders and Comorbidity in Suicide," American Journal of Psychiatry, Vol. 150, No. 6, June 1993, pp. 935–940.

Hepburn, L., M. Miller, D. Azrael, and D. Hemenway, "The US Gun Stock: Results from the 2004 National Firearms Survey," Injury Prevention, Vol. 13, No. 1, February 2007, pp. 15–19.

Hibbard, M. R., S. Uysal, M. Sliwinski, and W. A. Gordon, "Undiagnosed Health Issues in Individuals with Traumatic Brain Injury Living in the Community," Journal of Head Trauma Rehabilitation, Vol. 13, No. 4, August 1998, pp. 47–57.

Hilton, Susan M., David B. Service, Valerie A. Stander, Aaron D. Werbel, and Bonnie R. Chavez, *Department of the Navy Suicide Incident Report (DONSIR): Summary of 1999–2007 Findings*, U.S. Marine Corps, report 09-15, 2009.

Hoge, Charles W., Jennifer L. Auchterlonie, and Charles S. Milliken, "Mental Health Problems, Use of Mental Health Services, and Attrition from Military Service After Returning from Deployment to Iraq or Afghanistan," *Journal of the American Medical Association*, Vol. 295, No. 9, March 1, 2006, pp. 1023–1032.

Hoge, Charles W., Carl A. Castro, Stephen C. Messer, Dennis McGurk, Dave I. Cotting, and Robert L. Koffman, "Combat Duty in Iraq and Afghanistan, Mental Health Problems, and Barriers to Care," *New England Journal of Medicine*, Vol. 351, No. 1, July 1, 2004, pp. 13–22.

Hoge, Charles W., Dennis McGurk, Jeffrey L. Thomas, Anthony L. Cox, Charles C. Engel, and Carl A. Castro, "Mild Traumatic Brain Injury in U.S. Soldiers Returning from Iraq," *New England Journal of Medicine*, Vol. 359, No. 5, January 31, 2008, pp. 453–463.

Hourani, L. L., G. Warrack, and P. A. Coben, "A Demographic Analysis of Suicide Among U.S. Navy Personnel," *Suicide and Life-Threatening Behavior*, Vol. 29, No. 4, Winter 1999, pp. 365–375.

Høyer, G., and E. Lund, "Suicide Among Women Related to Number of Children in Marriage," *Archives of General Psychiatry*, Vol. 50, No. 2, February 1993, pp. 134–137.

HQMC—*see* Headquarters U.S. Marine Corps.

Insel, Beverly J., and Madelyn S. Gould, "Impact of Modeling on Adolescent Suicidal Behavior," *Psychiatric Clinics of North America*, Vol. 31, No. 2, June 2008, pp. 293–316.

Institute of Medicine, Committee on Crossing the Quality Chasm: Adaptation to Mental Health and Addictive Disorders, *Improving the Quality of Health Care for Mental and Substance-Use Conditions*, Washington, D.C.: National Academies Press, 2006. As of March 8, 2010: http://www.nap.edu/catalog/11470.html

IOM—*see* Institute of Medicine.

Isometsä, E. T., and J. K. Lönnqvist, "Suicide Attempts Preceding Completed Suicide," *British Journal of Psychiatry*, Vol. 173, December 1998, pp. 531–535.

Jacobson, Isabel G., Margaret A. K. Ryan, Tomoko I. Hooper, Tyler C. Smith, Paul J. Amoroso, Edward J. Boyko, Gary D. Gackstetter, Timothy S. Wells, and Nicole S. Bell, "Alcohol Use and Alcohol-Related Problems Before and After Military Combat Deployment," *Journal of the American Medical Association*, Vol. 300, No. 6, August 13, 2008, pp. 663–675.

Jobes, David A., Steven A. Wong, Amy K. Conrad, John F. Drozd, and Tracy Neal-Walden, "The Collaborative Assessment and Management of Suicidality Versus Treatment as Usual: A Retrospective Study with Suicidal Outpatients," *Suicide and Life-Threatening Behavior*, Vol. 35, No. 5, October 2005, pp. 483–497.

Joe, Sean, Silvia Sara Canetto, and Daniel Romer, "Advancing Prevention Research on the Role of Culture in Suicide Prevention," *Suicide and Life-Threatening Behavior*, Vol. 38, No. 3, June 2008, pp. 354–362.

Joe, Sean, and Mark S. Kaplan, "Suicide Among African American Men," *Suicide and Life-Threatening Behavior*, Vol. 31, No. 1, Suppl., March 2001, pp. 106–121.

Joiner, Thomas E., *Why People Die by Suicide*, Cambridge, Mass.: Harvard University Press, 2005.

Joiner, Thomas E., Jeremy W. Pettit, Rheeda L. Walker, Zachary R. Voelz, Jacqueline Cruz, M. David Rudd, and David I. Lester, "Perceived Burdensomeness and Suicidality: Two Studies on the Suicide Notes of Those Attempting and Those Completing Suicide," *Journal of Social and Clinical Psychology*, Vol. 21, No. 5, 2001, pp. 531–545.

Joiner, Thomas E. Jr., and M. David Rudd, "Intensity and Duration of Suicidal Crisis Vary as a Function of Previous Suicide Attempts and Negative Life Events," *Journal of Consulting and Clinical Psychology*, Vol. 68, No. 5, October 2000, pp. 909–916.

Joiner, Thomas E. Jr., Robert A. Steer, Gregory Brown, Aaron T. Beck, Jeremy W. Pettit, and M. David Rudd, "Worst-Point Suicidal Plans: A Dimension of Suicidality Predictive of Past Suicide Attempts and Eventual Death by Suicide," *Behaviour Research and Therapy*, Vol. 41, No. 12, December 2003, pp. 1469–1480.

Joiner, Thomas E. Jr., and Kimberly A. Van Orden, "The Interpersonal-Psychological Theory of Suicidal Behavior Indicates Specific and Crucial Psychotherapeutic Targets," *International Journal of Cognitive Therapy*, Vol. 1, No. 1, 2008, pp. 80–89.

JP 1-02—*see* U.S. Joint Chiefs of Staff (2001 [2009]).

Jumper, Gen. John P., Chief of Staff, U.S. Air Force, "Post-Suicide Assessment Process," memorandum for chiefs of staff, all major commands, field operating agencies, direct reporting units, and Air Force Reserve, October 7, 2002a.

———, "Policy for Investigative Interviews," memorandum for all major commands, field operating agencies, direct reporting units, and chief of staff, Air Force/Reserves, November 26, 2002b. As of March 5, 2010:
http://afspp.afms.mil/idc/groups/public/documents/afms/ctb_014097.pdf

Kalafat, J., Madelyn S. Gould, J. L. Munfakh, and Marjorie Kleinman, "An Evaluation of Crisis Hotline Outcomes, Part 1: Nonsuicidal Crisis Callers," *Suicide and Life-Threatening Behavior*, Vol. 37, No. 3, June 2007, pp. 322–337.

Karney, Benjamin R., Rajeev Ramchand, Karen Chan Osilla, Leah Barnes Caldarone, and Rachel M. Burns, "Predicting the Immediate and Long-Term Consequences of Post-Traumatic Stress Disorder, Depression, and Traumatic Brain Injury in Veterans of Operation Enduring Freedom and Operation Iraqi Freedom," in Terri Tanielian and Lisa H. Jaycox, eds., *Invisible Wounds of War: Psychological and Cognitive Injuries, Their Consequences, and Services to Assist Recovery*, Santa Monica, Calif.: RAND Corporation, MG-720-CCF, 2008, pp. 119–166. As of March 8, 2010:
http://www.rand.org/pubs/monographs/MG720/

Kellermann, A. L., F. P. Rivara, G. Somes, D. T. Reay, J. Francisco, J. G. Banton, J. Prodzinski, C. Fligner, and B. B. Hackman, "Suicide in the Home in Relation to Gun Ownership," *New England Journal of Medicine*, Vol. 327, No. 7, August 13, 1992, pp. 467–472.

Kelly, T. M., and J. J. Mann, "Validity of DSM-III-R Diagnosis by Psychological Autopsy: A Comparison with Clinician Ante-Mortem Diagnosis," *Acta Psychiatrica Scandinavica*, Vol. 94, No. 5, November 1996, pp. 337–343.

Kessler, R. C., P. A. Berglund, M. L. Bruce, J. R. Koch, E. M. Laska, P. J. Leaf, R. W. Manderscheid, R. A. Rosenheck, E. E. Walters, and P. S. Wang, "The Prevalence and Correlates of Untreated Serious Mental Illness," *Health Services Research*, Vol. 36, No. 6, Pt. 1, December 2001, pp. 987–1007.

Kessler, R. C., G. Borges, and E. E. Walters, "Prevalence of and Risk Factors for Lifetime Suicide Attempts in the National Comorbidity Survey," *Archives of General Psychiatry*, Vol. 56, No. 5, July 1999, pp. 617–626.

Kessler, R. C., G. Downey, J. R. Milavsky, and H. Stipp, "Clustering of Teenage Suicides After Television News Stories About Suicides: A Reconsideration," *American Journal of Psychiatry*, Vol. 145, 1988, pp. 1379–1383.

Kessler, R. C., G. Downey, H. Stipp, and J. R. Milavsky, "Network Television News Stories About Suicide and Short-Term Changes in Total U.S. Suicides," *Journal of Nervous and Mental Disease*, Vol. 177, No. 9, September 1989, pp. 551–555.

Kindt, Lt. Col. Michael, Air Force Suicide Prevention Program Manager, "Talking Paper on 2008 AF Suicide Trends," July 2009.

King, Keith A., and Judie Smith, "Project SOAR: A Training Program to Increase School Counselors' Knowledge and Confidence Regarding Suicide Prevention and Intervention," *Journal of School Health*, Vol. 70, No. 10, December 2000, pp. 402–407.

Knox, Kerry L., David A. Litts, G. Wayne Talcott, Jill Catalano Feig, and Eric D. Caine, "Risk of Suicide and Related Adverse Outcomes After Exposure to a Suicide Prevention Programme in the US Air Force: Cohort Study," *BMJ*, Vol. 327, No. 7428, December 13, 2003, p. 1376.

Kraemer, H. C., A. E. Kazdin, D. R. Offord, R. C. Kessler, P. S. Jensen, and D. J. Kupfer, "Coming to Terms with the Terms of Risk," *Archives of General Psychiatry*, Vol. 54, No. 4, April 1997, pp. 337–343.

Kraft, Heidi, and CAPT Richard Westphal, "Rule Number 2 and the Caregiver Occupational Stress Control Program," *Caregiver Operational Stress Control Training*, briefing slides provided to the authors, undated.

Kung, H. C., J. L. Pearson, and R. Wei, "Substance Use, Firearm Availability, Depressive Symptoms, and Mental Health Service Utilization Among White and African American Suicide Decedents Aged 15 to 64 Years," *Annals of Epidemiology*, Vol. 15, No. 8, September 2005, pp. 614–621.

Landstuhl Regional Medical Center Public Affairs, "Chief Outlines Comprehensive Soldier Fitness at Landstuhl," U.S. Army, September 30, 2009. As of March 8, 2010:
http://www.army.mil/-news/2009/09/30/
28086-chief-outlines-comprehensive-soldier-fitness-at-landstuhl/index.html

Leenaars, A. A., B. Yang, and D. Lester, "The Effect of Domestic and Economic Stress on Suicide Rates in Canada and the United States," *Journal of Clinical Psychology*, Vol. 49, No. 6, November 1993, pp. 918–921.

Leitner, Maria, Wally Barr, and Lindsay Hobby, *Effectiveness of Interventions to Prevent Suicide and Suicidal Behaviour: A Systematic Review*, Edinburgh, Scotland: Scottish Government Social Research, 2008.

Lichte, Lt. Gen. Arthur J., Assistant Vice Chief of Staff and Director, Air Force Staff, Headquarters U.S. Air Force, "Lessons Learned from AF Suicides," memorandum for all major commands, field operating agencies, and direct reporting units, June 6, 2007. As of March 8, 2010:
http://afspp.afms.mil/idc/groups/public/documents/afms/ctb_082897.pdf

Linehan, Marsha M., Katherine Anne Comtois, Milton Z. Brown, Heidi L. Heard, and Amy Wagner, "Suicide Attempt Self-Injury Interview (SASII): Development, Reliability, and Validity of a Scale to Assess Suicide Attempts and Intentional Self-Injury," *Psychological Assessment*, Vol. 18, No. 3, September 2006, pp. 303–312.

Linehan, Marsha M., Katherine Anne Comtois, Angela M. Murray, Milton Z. Brown, Robert J. Gallop, Heidi L. Heard, Kathryn E. Korslynd, Darren A. Tutek, Sarah K. Reynolds, and Noam Lindenboim, "Two-Year Randomized Controlled Trial and Follow-Up of Dialectical Behavior Therapy vs Therapy by Experts for Suicidal Behaviors and Borderline Personality Disorder," *Archives of General Psychiatry*, Vol. 63, No. 7, July 2006, pp. 757–766.

Linehan, Marsha M., Shireen L. Rizvi, Stacy Shaw Welch, and Benjamin Page, "Psychiatric Aspects of Suicidal Behaviour: Personality Disorders," in Keith Hawton and Kees van Heeringen, eds., *The International Handbook of Suicide and Attempted Suicide*, New York: Wiley, 2000, pp. 147–178.

Litts, D. A., K. Moe, C. H. Roadman, R. Janke, and J. Miller, "Suicide Prevention Among Active Duty Air Force Personnel: United States, 1990–1999," *Morbidity and Mortality Weekly Report*, Vol. 48, No. 46, November 26, 1999, pp. 1053–1057.

Litz, Brett T., Charles C. Engel, Richard A. Bryant, and Anthony Papa, "A Randomized, Controlled Proof-of-Concept Trial of an Internet-Based, Therapist-Assisted Self-Management Treatment for Posttraumatic Stress Disorder," *American Journal of Psychiatry*, Vol. 164, No. 11, November 2007, pp. 1676–1683.

LivingWorks, "ASIST: Applied Suicide Intervention Skills Training," last updated March 15, 2010. As of March 16, 2010:
http://www.livingworks.net/AS.php

Loftus, Maj. Gen. Thomas J., Assistant Surgeon General for Health Care Operations, Office of the Surgeon General, Department of the Air Force, "Frontline Supervisor's Training: Assisting Airmen in Distress," memorandum for all major commands and security forces, February 28, 2008a. As of March 8, 2010:
http://airforcemedicine.afms.mil/idc/groups/public/documents/afms/ctb_091976.pdf

———, "AF Suicide Trends," memorandum for surgeons general, headquarters U.S. Air Force Academy, Air Combat Command, Air Force District of Washington, Air Education and Training Command, Air Force Materiel Command, Air Force Special Operations Command, Air Force Space Command, Air Mobility Command, Pacific Air Forces, U.S. Air Forces in Europe, Air Force Reserve Command, and Air National Guard, and U.S. Air Force Medical Operations Agency South, August 1, 2008b.

Luoma, Jason B., Catherine E. Martin, and Jane L. Pearson, "Contact with Mental Health and Primary Care Providers Before Suicide: A Review of the Evidence," *American Journal of Psychiatry*, Vol. 159, No. 6, June 2002, pp. 909–916.

Luoma, Jason B., and Jane L. Pearson, "Suicide and Marital Status in the United States, 1991–1996: Is Widowhood a Risk Factor?" *American Journal of Public Health*, Vol. 92, No. 9, September 2002, pp. 1518–1522.

MACE—*see* Martial Arts Center of Excellence.

MacMahon, Brian, and Thomas F. Pugh, "Suicide in the Widowed," *American Journal of Epidemiology*, Vol. 81, No. 1, January 1965, pp. 23–31.

Mahon, Martin J., John P. Tobin, Denis A. Cusack, Cecily Kelleher, and Kevin M. Malone, "Suicide Among Regular-Duty Military Personnel: A Retrospective Case-Control Study of Occupation-Specific Risk Factors for Workplace Suicide," *American Journal of Psychiatry*, Vol. 162, September 2005, pp. 1688–1696.

Mann, J. John, "A Current Perspective of Suicide and Attempted Suicide," *Annals of Internal Medicine*, Vol. 136, No. 4, February 19, 2002, pp. 302–311.

———, "The Medical Management of Depression," *New England Journal of Medicine*, Vol. 353, No. 17, October 27, 2005, pp. 1819–1834.

Mann, J. John, Christine Waternaux, Gretchen L. Haas, and Kevin M. Malone, "Toward a Clinical Model of Suicidal Behavior in Psychiatric Patients," *American Journal of Psychiatry*, Vol. 156, February 1999, pp. 181–189.

MARADMIN 134/09—*see* Commandant of the Marine Corps (2009a).

MARADMIN 147/08—*see* Commandant of the Marine Corps (2008).

MARADMIN 364/09—*see* Commandant of the Marine Corps (2009b).

MARADMIN 404/09—*see* Commandant of the Marine Corps (2009c).

MARADMIN 436/09—*see* Commandant of the Marine Corps (2009d).

MARADMIN 596/09—*see* Commandant of the Marine Corps (2009e).

Marine Corps Community Services, "Leaders Guide for Managing Marines in Distress," home page, undated (a). As of March 16, 2010:
http://www.usmc-mccs.org/leadersguide/

———, "Making the Critical Decision," video, undated (b). As of March 11, 2010:
http://www.usmc-mccs.org/downloads/suicide/making_the_critical_decision.mpeg

———, "Military Life: Suicide Prevention," last updated March 13, 2007a. As of March 12, 2010:
http://www.usmc-mccs.org/suicideprevent/

———, "NCO Training Course Resource Library," last updated March 13, 2007b. As of March 16, 2010:
http://www.usmc-mccs.org/suicideprevent/ncotrng.cfm?sid=ml&smid=9

———, "COSC Continuum and Decision Matrix," last updated March 13, 2007c. As of May 7, 2010:
http://www.usmc-mccs.org/cosc/coscContMatrixMarines.cfm

———, home page, last updated August 21, 2009. As of March 16, 2010:
http://www.usmc-mccs.org/

Marine Corps Manpower and Reserve Affairs, undated home page. As of March 16, 2010:
https://www.manpower.usmc.mil/portal/page?_pageid=278,1&_dad=portal&_schema=PORTAL

Martial Arts Center of Excellence, undated web page. As of March 16, 2010:
http://www.tecom.usmc.mil/mace/

Maxwell, Jessica, "Army Stands Down for Suicide Prevention Training," U.S. Army, February 26, 2009. As of March 8, 2010:
http://www.army.mil/-news/2009/02/26/17471-army-stands-down-for-suicide-prevention-training/

McAuliffe, Nora, and Lynda Perry, "Making It Safer: A Health Centre's Strategy for Suicide Prevention," *Psychiatric Quarterly*, Vol. 78, No. 4, December 2007, pp. 295–307.

MCCS—*see* Marine Corps Community Services.

McGinn, Gail H., Deputy Under Secretary of Defense (Plans), "Department of Defense Calendar Year 2008 Suicides," memorandum for the Secretary of Defense, July 2, 2009.

McKeown, Robert E., Steven P. Cuffe, and Richard M. Schulz, "US Suicide Rates by Age Group, 1970–2002: An Examination of Recent Trends," *American Journal of Public Health*, Vol. 96, No. 10, October 2006, pp. 1744–1751.

McMillan, Dean, Simon Gilbody, Emma Beresford, and Liz Neilly, "Can We Predict Suicide and Non-Fatal Self-Harm with the Beck Hopelessness Scale? A Meta-Analysis," *Psychological Medicine*, Vol. 37, No. 6, June 2007, pp. 769–778.

MCO 1510.89B—*see* Headquarters U.S. Marine Corps (2004).

MCO P1700.24B—*see* Headquarters U.S. Marine Corps (2001).

MCO P1700.27A—*see* Headquarters U.S. Marine Corps (1999a).

MCO P1700.29—*see* Headquarters U.S. Marine Corps (1999b).

MCO P3040.4E—*see* Headquarters U.S. Marine Corps (2003).

MCRP 6-11C—*see* U.S. Marine Corps and U.S. Department of the Army (2000).

Meehan, P. J., J. A. Lamb, L. E. Saltzman, and P. W. O'Carroll, "Attempted Suicide Among Young Adults: Progress Toward a Meaningful Estimate of Prevalence," *American Journal of Psychiatry*, Vol. 149, No. 1, January 1992, pp. 41–44.

Michel, Konrad, "Suicide Prevention and Primary Care," in Keith Hawton and Kees van Heeringen, eds., *The International Handbook of Suicide and Attempted Suicide*, New York: Wiley, 2000, pp. 661–674.

Military Pathways, undated home page. As of March 15, 2010:
http://mentalhealthscreening.org/military/

Miller, Matthew, Deborah Azrael, L. Hepburn, David Hemenway, and Steven J. Lippmann, "The Association Between Changes in Household Firearm Ownership and Rates of Suicide in the United States, 1981–2002," *Injury Prevention*, Vol. 12, No. 3, June 2006, pp. 178–182.

Miller, Matthew, Steven J. Lippmann, Deborah Azrael, and David Hemenway, "Household Firearm Ownership and Rates of Suicide Across the 50 United States," *Journal of Trauma*, Vol. 62, No. 4, April 2007, pp. 1029–1034; discussion pp. 1034–1025.

Miller, Michael Craig, Douglas G. Jacobs, and Thomas G. Gutheil, "Talisman or Taboo: The Controversy of the Suicide-Prevention Contract," *Harvard Review of Psychiatry*, Vol. 6, No. 2, July–August 1998, pp. 78–87.

Milliken, Charles S., Jennifer L. Auchterlonie, and Charles W. Hoge, "Longitudinal Assessment of Mental Health Problems Among Active and Reserve Component Soldiers Returning from the Iraq War," *Journal of the American Medical Association*, Vol. 298, No. 18, November 14, 2007, pp. 2141–2148.

Milstein, Robert L., and Scott F. Wetterhall, "Framework for Program Evaluation in Public Health," *Morbidity and Mortality Weekly Report Recommendations and Reports*, Vol. 48, No. RR11, September 17, 1999, pp. 1–40. As of March 8, 2010:
http://www.cdc.gov/mmwr/preview/mmwrhtml/rr4811a1.htm

Molnar, B. E., L. F. Berkman, and S. L. Buka, "Psychopathology, Childhood Sexual Abuse and Other Childhood Adversities: Relative Links to Subsequent Suicidal Behaviour in the US," *Psychological Medicine*, Vol. 31, No. 6, August 2001, pp. 965–977.

Morgan, H. G., E. M. Jones, and J. H. Owen, "Secondary Prevention of Non-Fatal Deliberate Self-Harm: The Green Card Study," *British Journal of Psychiatry*, Vol. 163, 1993, pp. 111–112.

Motto, Jerome A., and Alan G. Bostrom, "A Randomized Controlled Trial of Postcrisis Suicide Prevention," *Psychiatric Services*, Vol. 52, June 2001, pp. 828–833.

Mrazek, Patricia Beezley, and Robert J. Haggerty, eds., *Reducing Risks for Mental Disorders: Frontiers for Preventive Intervention Research*, Washington, D.C.: National Academy Press, 1994. As of March 8, 2010:
http://books.nap.edu/openbook.php?isbn=0309049393

Nash, William P., "Operational Stress Control and Readiness (OSCAR): The United States Marine Corps Initiative to Deliver Mental Health Services to Operating Forces," in *Human Dimensions in Military Operations: Military Leaders' Strategies for Addressing Stress and Psychological Support*, meeting proceedings RTO-MP-HFM-134, paper 25, Neuilly-sur-Seine, France, April 1, 2006, pp. 25-1–25-10. As of March 8, 2010:
http://handle.dtic.mil/100.2/ADA472703

National Research Council, Committee on the Youth Population and Military Recruitment, *Assessing Fitness for Military Enlistment: Physical, Medical, and Mental Health Standards*, Washington, D.C.: National Academies Press, 2006.

NAVADMIN 033/09—*see* Chief of Naval Operations (2009a).

NAVADMIN 122/09—*see* Chief of Naval Operations (2009b).

NAVADMIN 182/07—*see* Chief of Naval Operations (2007).

NAVADMIN 243/05—*see* Chief of Naval Operations (2005).

Naval Education and Training Command, "N@vy Knowledge Online," undated home page. As of March 16, 2010:
https://wwwa.nko.navy.mil/portal/home/

———, "Naval Education and Training Command," last updated November 9, 2009. As of March 16, 2010:
https://www.netc.navy.mil/

NAVPERS—*see* Navy Personnel Command.

Navy and Marine Corps Public Health Center, "Suicide Prevention: Presentations," last updated February 23, 2009a. As of March 11, 2010:
http://www.nmcphc.med.navy.mil/Healthy_Living/Psychological_Health/Suicide_Prevention/prevsuicide_presentations.aspx

———, "Operational and Combat Stress," last updated October 7, 2009b. As of March 8, 2010:
http://www.nmcphc.med.navy.mil/healthy_living/psychological_health/stress_management/operandcombatstress.aspx

Navy Medicine, undated home page. As of March 16, 2010:
http://www.med.navy.mil/bumed/Pages/default.aspx

Navy Personnel Command, *Navy Casualty Assistance Calls Officer (CACO) Program*, undated. As of November 20, 2009:
http://www.npc.navy.mil/NR/rdonlyres/3BB8B920-69C3-4A88-AF44-01EC5248BDE7/0/navyCACO.pdf

———, "Poster Downloads," last updated May 28, 2009. As of March 11, 2010:
http://www.npc.navy.mil/CommandSupport/SuicidePrevention/CommandLeaders/sp_posters.htm

———, "Suicide Prevention," last updated March 5, 2010a. As of March 11, 2010:
http://www.npc.navy.mil/CommandSupport/SuicidePrevention/

———, home page, last updated March 15, 2010b. As of March 16, 2010:
http://www.npc.navy.mil/channels

NETC—*see* Naval Education and Training Command.

Newell, C., K. Whittam, and Z. Uriell, *Behavioral Health Quick Poll*, Navy Personnel Research Studies and Technology, Bureau of Navy Personnel, 2009.

NMCPHC—*see* Navy and Marine Corps Public Health Center.

Norton, Ken, "Connect Suicide Prevention Project," paper presented at Joint Family Readiness Conference, Chicago, Ill., September 3, 2009.

Nutting, Paul A., Kaia Gallagher, Kim Riley, Suzanne White, W. Perry Dickinson, Neil Korsen, and Allen Dietrich, "Care Management for Depression in Primary Care Practice: Findings from the RESPECT-Depression Trial," *Annals of Family Medicine*, Vol. 6, 2008, pp. 30–37.

O'Carroll, P. W., A. L. Berman, R. W. Maris, E. K. Moscicki, B. L. Tanney, and M. M. Silverman, "Beyond the Tower of Babel: A Nomenclature for Suicidology," *Suicide and Life-Threatening Behavior*, Vol. 26, No. 3, Fall 1996, pp. 237–252.

O'Carroll, P. W., J. A. Mercy, and J. A. Steward, "CDC Recommendations for a Community Plan for the Prevention and Containment of Suicide Clusters," *Morbidity and Mortality Weekly Report*, Vol. 37, Suppl. 6, August 19, 1988, pp. 1–12. As of March 8, 2010: http://wonder.cdc.gov/wonder/prevguid/p0000214/p0000214.asp

Office of the Chief of Naval Operations, Department of the Navy, Suicide Prevention Program, Chief of Naval Operations instruction 1720.4A, August 4, 2009. As of March 8, 2010: http://www.nmcphc.med.navy.mil/downloads/healthyliv/SuicidePrevention/ SUICIDE_PREVENTION_OPNAV4AUG09.pdf

Oordt, Mark S., David A. Jobes, M. David Rudd, Vincent P. Fonseca, Christine N. Runyan, John B. Stea, Rick L. Campise, and G. Wayne Talcott, "Development of a Clinical Guide to Enhance Care for Suicidal Patients," *Professional Psychology: Research and Practice*, Vol. 36, No. 2, 2005, pp. 208–218.

OPNAVINST 1720.4A—*see* Office of the Chief of Naval Operations (2009).

Paolucci, Elizabeth Oddone, Mark L. Genuis, and Claudio Violato, "A Meta-Analysis of the Published Research on the Effects of Child Sexual Abuse," *Journal of Psychology*, Vol. 135, No. 1, 2001, pp. 17–36.

Paykel, Eugene S., Brigitte A. Prusoff, and Jerome K. Myers, "Suicide Attempts and Recent Life Events: A Controlled Comparison," *Archives of General Psychiatry*, Vol. 32, No. 3, March 1975, pp. 327–333.

Pearse, Lisa, "Numbers Count: Apples, Oranges and the Occasional Banana," Mortality Surveillance Division, Armed Forces Medical Examiner System, Armed Forces Institute of Pathology, undated briefing. As of March 8, 2010: http://www.ha.osd.mil/2008mspc/downloads/NumbersCount-PearseApr08-red_POST_Pearse.pdf

Pflanz, Steven, "Bullet Background Paper on Landing Gear," April 2008. As of November 20, 2009: http://airforcemedicine.afms.mil/idc/groups/public/documents/afms/ctb_095433.pdf

Phillips, D. P., and D. J. Paight, "The Impact of Televised Movies About Suicide: A Replicative Study," *New England Journal of Medicine*, Vol. 317, No. 13, September 24, 1987, pp. 809–811.

Pignone, Michael P., Bradley N. Gaynes, Jerry L. Rushton, Catherine Mills Burchell, C. Tracy Orleans, Cynthia D. Mulrow, and Kathleen N. Lohr, "Screening for Depression in Adults: A Summary of the Evidence for the U.S. Preventive Services Task Force," *Annals of Internal Medicine*, Vol. 136, No. 10, May 21, 2002, pp. 765–776.

Pirkis, Jane, "Suicide and the Media," *Psychiatry*, Vol. 8, No. 7, July 2009, pp. 269–271.

Pirkis, Jane, R. Warwick Blood, Annette Beautrais, Philip Burgess, and Jaelea Skehan, "Media Guidelines on the Reporting of Suicide," *Crisis*, Vol. 27, No. 2, 2006, pp. 82–87.

Platt, S., "Unemployment and Suicidal Behaviour: A Review of the Literature," *Social Science and Medicine*, Vol. 19, No. 2, 1984, pp. 93–115.

Platt, S., U. Bille-Brahe, A. Kerkhof, A. Schmidtke, T. Bjerke, P. Crepet, D. De Leo, C. Haring, J. Lonnqvist, K. Michel, et al., "Parasuicide in Europe: The WHO/EURO Multicentre Study on Parasuicide, I: Introduction and Preliminary Analysis for 1989," *Acta Psychiatrica Scandinavia*, Vol. 85, No. 2, February 1992, pp. 97–104.

Pollock, L. R., and J. M. G. Williams, "Problem-Solving in Suicide Attempters," *Psychological Medicine*, Vol. 34, No. 1, January 2004, pp. 163–167.

Posner, Kelly, Maria A. Oquendo, Madelyn Gould, Barbara Stanley, and Mark Davies, "Columbia Classification Algorithm of Suicide Assessment (C-CASA): Classification of Suicidal Events in the FDA's Pediatric Suicidal Risk Analysis of Antidepressants," *American Journal of Psychiatry*, Vol. 164, July 2007, pp. 1035–1043.

Public Law 90-618, Gun Control Act of 1968, October 22, 1968.

Public Law 104-208, Making Omnibus Consolidated Appropriations for the Fiscal Year Ending September 30, 1997, and for Other Purposes, Section 658, Gun Ban for Individuals Convicted of a Misdemeanor Crime of Domestic Violence. As of March 15, 2010:
http://frwebgate.access.gpo.gov/cgi-bin/
getdoc.cgi?dbname=104_cong_public_laws&docid=f:publ208.104

Public Law 108-355, Garrett Lee Smith Memorial Act, October 24, 2004.

Public Law 110-28, U.S. Troop Readiness, Veterans' Care, Katrina Recovery, and Iraq Accountability Appropriations Act, May 25, 2007. As of March 15, 2010:
http://frwebgate.access.gpo.gov/cgi-bin/
getdoc.cgi?dbname=110_cong_public_laws&docid=f:publ028.110

Raue, P. J., E. L. Brown, B. S. Meyers, H. C. Schulberg, and M. L. Bruce, "Does Every Allusion to Possible Suicide Require the Same Response?" *Journal of Family Practice*, Vol. 55, No. 7, July 2006, pp. 605–612.

RESPECT-Mil, undated home page. As of March 16, 2010:
http://www.pdhealth.mil/respect-mil/index1.asp

Roeder, K. T., M. A. Valenstein, J. H. Forman, H. M. Walters, M. Kulkarni, and J. K. Travis, "Acceptability of Interventions to Delay Gun Access for VA Patients at High Risk for Suicide," paper presented at American Association of Suicidology Annual Conference, San Francisco, Calif., April 2009.

Rose, S. C., J. Bisson, R. Churchill, and S. Wessely, "Psychological Debriefing for Preventing Post Traumatic Stress Disorder (PTSD)," *Cochrane Database of Systematic Reviews*, No. 2, article CD000560, 2002.

Rotheram-Borus, M. J., J. Piacentini, C. Cantwell, T. R. Belin, and J. Song, "The 18-Month Impact of an Emergency Room Intervention for Adolescent Female Suicide Attempters," *Journal of Consulting and Clinical Psychology*, Vol. 68, No. 6, December 2000, pp. 1081–1093.

Rowan, Anderson B., and Rick L. Campise, "A Multisite Study of Air Force Outpatient Behavioral Health Treatment-Seeking Patterns and Career Impact," *Military Medicine*, Vol. 171, No. 11, November 2006, pp. 1123–1127.

Roy, A., "Suicidal Behavior in Twins: A Replication," *Journal of Affective Disorders*, Vol. 66, No. 1, September 2001, pp. 71–74.

RTI International, "Department of Defense Lifestyle Assessment Program (DLAP)," last updated January 16, 2008. As of November 17, 2009:
http://dlap.rti.org/

Rudd, M. David, "Cognitive Therapy for Suicidality: An Integrative, Comprehensive, and Practical Approach to Conceptualization," *Journal of Contemporary Psychotherapy*, Vol. 34, No. 1, March 2004, pp. 59–72.

Rudd, M. David, M. Hasan Rajab, and P. Fred Dahm, "Problem-Solving Appraisal in Suicide Ideators and Attempters," *American Journal of Orthopsychiatry*, Vol. 58, No. 1, January 1994, pp. 136–149.

Russo, C. Allison, Pamela L. Owens, and Megan M. Hambrick, *Violence-Related Stays in U.S. Hospitals, 2005*, Rockville, Md.: Agency for Healthcare Research and Quality, statistical brief 48, March 2008. As of March 8, 2010:
http://www.hcup-us.ahrq.gov/reports/statbriefs/sb48.pdf

Rutz, W., L. von Knorring, and J. Wålinder, "Frequency of Suicide on Gotland After Systematic Postgraduate Education of General Practitioners," *Acta Psychiatrica Scandinavica*, Vol. 80, No. 2, August 1989, pp. 151–154.

SAMHSA—*see* Substance Abuse and Mental Health Services Administration.

Santa Mina, E. E., and R. M. Gallop, "Childhood Sexual and Physical Abuse and Adult Self-Harm and Suicidal Behaviour: A Literature Review," *Canadian Journal of Psychiatry*, Vol. 43, No. 8, October 1998, pp. 793–800.

Santelli, John S., Audrey Smith Rogers, Walter D. Rosenfeld, Robert H. DuRant, Nancy Dubler, Madlyn Morreale, Abigail English, Sheryl Lyss, Yolanda Wimberly, and Anna Schissel, "Guidelines for Adolescent Health Research: A Position Paper of the Society for Adolescent Medicine," *Journal of Adolescent Health*, Vol. 33, No. 5, November 2003, pp. 396–409.

Sareen, J., T. Houlahan, B. J. Cox, and G. J. Asmundson, "Anxiety Disorders Associated with Suicidal Ideation and Suicide Attempts in the National Comorbidity Survey," *Journal of Nervous and Mental Disease*, Vol. 193, No. 7, July 2005, pp. 450–454.

Schell, Terry L., and Grant N. Marshall, "Survey of Individuals Previously Deployed for OEF/OIF," in Terri Tanielian and Lisa H. Jaycox, eds., *Invisible Wounds of War: Psychological and Cognitive Injuries, Their Consequences, and Services to Assist Recovery*, Santa Monica, Calif.: RAND Corporation, MG-720-CCF, 2008, pp. 87–115. As of March 8, 2010:
http://www.rand.org/pubs/monographs/MG720/

Schoenbaum, M., R. Heinssen, and J. L. Pearson, "Opportunities to Improve Interventions to Reduce Suicidality: Civilian 'Best Practices' for Army Consideration," Bethesda, Md.: National Institute of Mental Health, 2009.

Schulsinger, F., S. S. Kety, D. Rosenthal, and P. H. Wender, "A Family Study of Suicide," in Mogens Schou and Erik Strömgren, eds., *Origin, Prevention, and Treatment of Affective Disorders*, London: Academic Press, 1979, pp. 277–287.

Shaffer, D., M. Scott, H. Wilcox, C. Maslow, R. Hicks, C. P. Lucas, R. Garfinkel, and S. Greenwald, "The Columbia Suicide Screen: Validity and Reliability of a Screen for Youth Suicide and Depression," *Journal of the American Academy of Child and Adolescent Psychiatry*, Vol. 43, No. 1, January 2004, pp. 71–79.

Sheftick, Gary, "Interactive DVD Among New Tools to Prevent Suicides," U.S. Army, September 2, 2008. As of March 8, 2010:
http://www.army.mil/-news/2008/09/03/12096-interactive-dvd-among-new-tools-to-prevent-suicides/

Silverman, M. M., A. L. Berman, N. D. Sanddal, P. W. O'Carroll, and T. E. Joiner, "Rebuilding the Tower of Babel: A Revised Nomenclature for the Study of Suicide and Suicidal Behaviors, Part 2: Suicide-Related Ideations, Communications, and Behaviors," *Suicide and Life-Threatening Behavior*, Vol. 37, No. 3, June 2007, pp. 264–277.

Simon, Robert I., "Gun Safety Management with Patients at Risk for Suicide," *Suicide and Life-Threatening Behavior*, Vol. 37, No. 5, October 2007, pp. 518–526.

Simpson, Grahame, and Robyn Tate, "Suicidality After Traumatic Brain Injury: Demographic, Injury and Clinical Correlates," *Psychological Medicine*, Vol. 32, No. 4, 2002, pp. 687–697.

————, "Clinical Features of Suicide Attempts After Traumatic Brain Injury," *Journal of Nervous and Mental Disease*, Vol. 193, No. 10, October 2005, pp. 680–685.

Smith, Tyler C., Margaret A. K. Ryan, Deborah L. Wingard, Donald J. Slymen, James F. Sallis, and Donna Kritz-Silverstein, "New Onset and Persistent Symptoms of Post-Traumatic Stress Disorder Self Reported After Deployment and Combat Exposures: Prospective Population Based US Military Cohort Study," *British Medical Journal*, Vol. 336, No. 7640, Febrary 16, 2008, pp. 366–371.

SRMSO—*see* Suicide Risk Management and Surveillance Office.

Stack, S., "A Reanalysis of the Impact of Non Celebrity Suicides," *Social Psychiatry and Psychiatric Epidemiology*, Vol. 25, No. 5, September 1990, pp. 269–273.

Stanley, Barbara, and Gregory K. Brown, *Safety Plan Treatment Manual to Reduce Suicide Risk: Veteran Version*, Washington, D.C.: U.S. Department of Veterans Affairs, 2008. As of March 8, 2010:
http://www.mentalhealth.va.gov/MENTALHEALTH/College/docs/
VA_Safety_planning_manual.doc

Statham, D. J., A. C. Heath, P. A. F. Madden, K. K. Bucholz, L. Bierut, S. H. Dinwiddie, W. S. Slutske, M. P. Dunne, and N. G. Martin, "Suicidal Behaviour: An Epidemiological and Genetic Study," *Psychological Medicine*, Vol. 28, 1998, pp. 839–855.

Strong Bonds, undated home page. As of March 16, 2010:
http://www.strongbonds.org/skins/strongbonds/display.aspx

Substance Abuse and Mental Health Services Administration, "Screening, Brief Intervention, and Referral to Treatment," undated web page. As of March 10, 2010:
http://sbirt.samhsa.gov/

————, Office of Applied Studies, *Suicidal Thoughts and Behaviors Among Adults*, Rockville, Md., September 17, 2009. As of March 8, 2010:
http://www.oas.samhsa.gov/2k9/165/SuicideHTML.pdf

————, "NREPP: SAMHSA's National Registry of Evidence-Based Programs and Practices," last updated February 18, 2010. As of March 11, 2010:
http://www.nrepp.samhsa.gov/

Suicide Prevention Resource Center Training Institute, "Assessing and Managing Suicide Risk: Core Competencies for Mental Health Professionals," undated web page. As of November 20, 2009:
http://www.sprc.org/traininginstitute/amsr/clincomp.asp

Suicide Risk Management and Surveillance Office, Army Behavioral Health Technology Office, Madigan Army Medical Center, *Army Suicide Event Report (ASER) Calendar Year 2006*, Tacoma, Wash., c. 2007.

————, *Army Suicide Event Report (ASER) Calendar Year 2007*, Tacoma, Wash., c. 2008.

Suominen, Kirsi, Erkki Isometsä, Jaana Suokas, Jari Haukka, Kalle Achte, and Jouko Lönnqvist, "Completed Suicide After a Suicide Attempt: A 37-Year Follow-Up Study," *American Journal of Psychiatry*, Vol. 161, No. 3, March 2004, pp. 562–563.

Sutton, BG Loree K., U.S. Army, Director, Defense Centers of Excellence for Psychological Health and Traumatic Brain Injury, prepared statement before the Senate Armed Services Committee, Subcommittee on Personnel, March 18, 2009. As of March 8, 2010:
http://www.senate.gov/~armed_services/statemnt/2009/March/Sutton%2003-18-09.pdf

Tanielian, Terri, Lisa H. Jaycox, Terry L. Schell, Grant N. Marshall, and Mary E. Vaiana, "Treating the Invisible Wounds of War: Conclusions and Recommendations," in Terri Tanielian and Lisa H. Jaycox, eds., *Invisible Wounds of War: Psychological and Cognitive Injuries, Their Consequences, and Services to Assist Recovery*, Santa Monica, Calif.: RAND Corporation, MG-720-CCF, 2008, pp. 431–453. As of March 8, 2010:
http://www.rand.org/pubs/monographs/MG720/

Teasdale, T. W., and A. W. Engberg, "Suicide After Traumatic Brain Injury: A Population Study," *Journal of Neurology, Neurosurgery and Psychiatry*, Vol. 71, No. 4, 2001, pp. 436–440.

TECOM—*see* U.S. Marine Corps Training and Education Command.

Thompson, Elaine Adams, and Leona L. Eggert, "Using the Suicide Risk Screen to Identify Suicidal Adolescents Among Potential High School Dropouts," *Journal of the American Academy of Child and Adolescent Psychiatry*, Vol. 38, No. 12, December 1999, pp. 1506–1514.

Thompson, Mark, "America's Medicated Army," *Time*, June 5, 2008. As of March 8, 2010:
http://www.time.com/time/nation/article/0,8599,1811858,00.html

Torsch, V., "Psychological Health Outreach Program," undated briefing slides provided to the authors.

TRADOC PAM 600-22—*see* Headquarters Department of the Army (2005).

Tsuang, M. T., R. F. Woolson, and J. A. Fleming, "Premature Deaths in Schizophrenia and Affective Disorders: An Analysis of Survival Curves and Variables Affecting the Shortened Survival," *Archives of General Psychiatry*, Vol. 37, No. 9, September 1980, pp. 979–983.

Uniform Code of Military Justice, Subchapter III, Non-Judicial Punishment, 815, Article 15, Commanding Officer's Non-Judicial Punishment. As of March 11, 2010:
http://www.au.af.mil/au/awc/awcgate/
ucmj.htm#SUBCHAPTER III. NON-JUDICIAL PUNISHMENT

———, Subchapter VI, Pre-Trial Procedure, 830, Article 30, Charges and Specifications. As of March 11, 2010:
http://www.au.af.mil/au/awc/awcgate/ucmj.htm#SUBCHAPTER VI. PRE-TRIAL PROCEDURE

Unützer, J., W. Katon, C. M. Callahan, J. W. Williams Jr., E. Hunkeler, L. Harpole, M. Hoffing, R. D. Della Penna, P. H. Noël, E. H. Lin, P. A. Areán, M. T. Hegel, L. Tang, T. R. Belin, S. Oishi, and C. Langston, "Collaborative Care Management of Late-Life Depression in the Primary Care Setting: A Randomized Controlled Trial," *Journal of the American Medical Association*, Vol. 288, No. 22, December 11, 2002, pp. 2836–2845.

U.S. Air Force, "Air Force Suicide Prevention Program," undated website. As of March 11, 2010:
http://afspp.afms.mil/idc/groups/public/documents/webcontent/knowledgejunction.hcst?
functionalarea=AFSuicidePreventionPrgm&doctype=subpage&docname=CTB_018094&
incbanner=0

U.S. Army, "Comprehensive Soldier Fitness: Strong Minds, Strong Bodies," undated web page. As of March 11, 2010:
http://www.army.mil/csf/

———, *Guide to the Prevention of Suicide and Self-Destructive Behavior*, Washington, D.C., Department of the Army pamphlet 600-70, 1985.

U.S. Army Center for Health Promotion and Preventive Medicine, "Army's ACE Suicide Intervention Program: Train the Trainers Manual," January 31, 2008.

———, home page, last updated December 11, 2009. As of March 11, 2010:
http://chppm-www.apgea.army.mil/

————, "USACHPPM Directorate of Health Promotion and Wellness," last updated January 2010. As of March 15, 2010:
http://chppm-www.apgea.army.mil/dhpw/

U.S. Army Human Resources Policy Directorate, "Intervention Training Scenarios," September 3, 2008.

U.S. Army Medical Department, "Combat Stress Control," last modified June 25, 2008. As of November 21, 2009:
http://www.armymedicine.army.mil/about/tl/factscombatstresscontrol.html

————, "Mental Health Reports (OIF)," last modified November 24, 2009. As of March 16, 2010:
http://www.armymedicine.army.mil/reports/mhat/mhat.html

————, "Resilience Training (Formerly Battlemind)," last modified February 22, 2010. As of March 16, 2010:
https://www.resilience.army.mil/

U.S. Army Public Health Command (Provisional), home page, last updated April 7, 2010. As of March 30, 2010:
http://usachppm.apgea.army.mil/APHC/

U.S. Census Bureau, data set generated by Rajeev Ramchand using American Factfinder, February 3, 2010.

U.S. Department of the Air Force, *Frontline Supervisors Training: Manual for Instructors and Students*, undated. As of March 8, 2010:
http://airforcemedicine.afms.mil/idc/groups/public/documents/afms/ctb_091855.pdf

————, Medical: Mental Health, Confidentiality, and Military Law, Air Force instruction 44-109, March 1, 2000. As of March 8, 2010:
http://www.af.mil/shared/media/epubs/AFI44-109.pdf

————, *The Air Force Suicide Prevention Program: A Description of Program Initiatives and Outcomes*, Air Force pamphlet 44-160, April 2001. As of March 8, 2010:
http://afspp.afms.mil/idc/groups/public/documents/afms/ctb_056459.pdf

————, Medical: Suicide and Violence Prevention Education and Training, Air Force instruction 44-154, January 3, 2003. As of March 8, 2010:
http://www.af.mil/shared/media/epubs/AFI44-154.pdf

————, Health Services Inspection Guide, 2006a.

————, Patient Administration Functions, Air Force instruction 41-210, March 22, 2006b (incorporating change 2, November 29, 2010). As of January 4, 2011:
http://www.af.mil/shared/media/epubs/AFI41-210.pdf

————, Medical: Traumatic Stress Response, Air Force instruction 44-153, March 31, 2006c. As of March 12, 2010:
http://www.af.mil/shared/media/epubs/AFI44-153.pdf

————, Specialty Management: Community Action Information Board and Integrated Delivery System, Air Force instruction 90-501, August 31, 2006d. As of March 8, 2010:
http://www.af.mil/shared/media/epubs/AFI90-501.pdf

U.S. Department of the Army, *Leaders' Manual for Combat Stress Control*, Washington, D.C., Army field manual 22-51, September 29, 1994.

———, "Army Suicide Prevention Program," *2008 Army Posture Statement*, c. 2008a. As of March 8, 2010:
http://www.army.mil/aps/08/information_papers/sustain/Army_Suicide_Prevention_Program.html

———, "Pre-Deployment Battlemind for Warriors," PSB04001/1, May 22, 2008b.

———, *Army Suicide Prevention Program: Intervention Training Scenarios*, September 3, 2008c. As of March 11, 2010:
http://www.armyg1.army.mil/hr/suicide/docs/
Suicide%20Prevention%20Training%20Scenarios%20Q%20&%20A.pdf

———, "Army Campaign Plan for Health Promotion, Risk Reduction and Suicide Prevention," *2010 Army Posture Statement*, updated January 5, 2010. As of April 8, 2010:
https://secureweb2.hqda.pentagon.mil/vdas_armyposturestatement/2010/information_papers/Army_
Campaign_Plan_for_Health_Promotion,_Risk_Reduction_and_Suicide_Prevention.asp

U.S. Department of Defense, *Demographics 2007: Profile of the Military Community*, undated. As of March 8, 2010:
http://www.militaryonesource.com/MOS/ServiceProviders/
2007DemographicsProfileoftheMilitaryCommuni.aspx

———, Post-Deployment Health Assessment (PDHA), form DD2796, January 1, 2008. As of March 8, 2010:
http://www.dtic.mil/whs/directives/infomgt/forms/forminfo/forminfopage2347.html

———, "DoD Establishes Suicide Prevention Task Force," news release, 668-09, August 31, 2009a. As of March 11, 2010:
http://www.defense.gov/releases/release.aspx?releaseid=12941

———, "The Army's Suicide Prevention Efforts," news transcript, November 17, 2009b. As of November 20, 2009:
http://www.defenselink.mil/transcripts/transcript.aspx?transcriptid=4513

U.S. Department of Health and Human Services, Substance Abuse and Mental Health Services Administration, National Registry of Evidence-Based Programs and Practices, "TeenScreen," last updated March 18, 2010. As of November 17, 2009:
http://www.nrepp.samhsa.gov/programfulldetails.asp?PROGRAM_ID=108

U.S. Joint Chiefs of Staff, *Department of Defense Dictionary of Military and Associated Terms*, Washington, D.C., joint publication 1-02, April 12, 2001, as amended through October 31, 2009. As of March 8, 2010:
http://purl.access.gpo.gov/GPO/LPS14106

U.S. Marine Corps, and U.S. Department of the Army, *Combat Stress*, Washington, D.C., Marine Corps reference publication 6-11C, Army field manual 90-44/6-22.5, Navy Tactics, Techniques, and Procedures 1-15M, 2000. As of March 8, 2010:
http://www.au.af.mil/au/awc/awcgate/usmc/mcrp611c.pdf

U.S. Marine Corps Forces Reserve, "Combat Operational Stress Control," undated web page. As of November 20, 2009:
http://www.marforres.usmc.mil/MFRHQ/COSC/default.asp

U.S. Marine Corps Training and Education Command, undated home page. As of March 15, 2010:
http://www.tecom.usmc.mil/

U.S. Navy, "Navy Personnel Urged to AID LIFE in Suicide Awareness, Prevention," story NNS051110-02, November 10, 2005. As of March 11, 2010:
http://www.navy.mil/search/display.asp?story_id=20602

U.S. Preventive Services Task Force, "Topic Index: A–Z," undated web page. As of November 17, 2009:
http://www.ahrq.gov/clinic/uspstf/uspstopics.htm

U.S. Public Health Service, *National Strategy for Suicide Prevention: Goals and Objectives for Action*, Rockville, Md.: U.S. Department of Health and Human Services, Public Health Service, 2001. As of March 8, 2010:
http://mentalhealth.samhsa.gov/publications/allpubs/SMA01-3517/

Vaiva, Guillame, François Ducrocq, Philippe Meyer, Daniel Mathieu, Alain Philippe, Christian Libersa, and Michel Goudemand, "Effect of Telephone Contact on Further Suicide Attempts in Patients Discharged from an Emergency Department: Randomised Controlled Study," *BMJ*, Vol. 332, No. 7552, May 27, 2006, pp. 1241–1245.

Vasterling, Jennifer J., Susan P. Proctor, Paul Amoroso, Robert Kane, Timothy Heeren, and Roberta F. White, "Neuropsychological Outcomes of Army Personnel Following Deployment to the Iraq War," *Journal of the American Medical Association*, Vol. 296, No. 5, August 2, 2006, pp. 519–529.

Warden, D., "Military TBI During the Iraq and Afghanistan Wars," *Journal of Head Trauma Rehabilitation*, Vol. 21, No. 5, September–October 2006, pp. 398–402.

Wasserman, I. M., "The Influence of Economic Business Cycles on United States Suicide Rates," *Suicide and Life-Threatening Behavior*, Vol. 14, No. 3, Fall 1984, pp. 143–156.

Wenzel, Amy, and Aaron T. Beck, "A Cognitive Model of Suicidal Behavior: Theory and Treatment," *Applied and Preventive Psychology*, Vol. 12, No. 4, October 2008, pp. 189–201.

Wenzel, Amy, Gregory K. Brown, and Aaron T. Beck, *Cognitive Therapy for Suicidal Patients: Scientific and Clinical Applications*, 1st ed., Washington, D.C.: American Psychological Association, 2009.

Werbel, CDR Aaron D., suicide-prevention program manager, Headquarters, Marine Corps (Manpower and Reserve Affairs), "Marine Corps Suicide Prevention Program (MCSPP): Update," November 2009.

Westphal, R., "Navy/Marine Corps TBI/PH Resilience Programs," Defense Centers of Excellence Warriors Resilience Conference, Fairfax, Va., 2008.

Wilcox, Holly C., Kenneth R. Conner, and Eric D. Caine, "Association of Alcohol and Drug Use Disorders and Completed Suicide: An Empirical Review of Cohort Studies," *Drug and Alcohol Dependence*, Vol. 76, Suppl. 1, December 7, 2004, pp. S11–S19.

Wilcox, Holly C., Sheppard G. Kellam, C. Hendricks Brown, Jeanne M. Poduska, Nicholas S. Ialongo, Wei Wang, and James C. Anthony, "The Impact of Two Universal Randomized First- and Second-Grade Classroom Interventions on Young Adult Suicide Ideation and Attempts," *Drug and Alcohol Dependence*, Vol. 95, Suppl. 1, June 1, 2008, pp. S60–S73.

Williams, Farah, Carli Hague, and Dewey G. Cornell, "Evaluation of Statewide Training in Student Suicide Prevention," Charlottesville, Va.: Virginia Youth Violence Project, undated.

Wyman, Peter A., C. Hendricks Brown, Jeff Inman, Wendi Cross, Karen Schmeelk-Cone, Jing Guo, and Juan B. Pena, "Randomized Trial of a Gatekeeper Program for Suicide Prevention: 1-Year Impact on Secondary School Staff," *Journal of Consulting and Clinical Psychology*, Vol. 76, No. 1, February 2008, pp. 104–115.

Ybarra, M. L., and W. W. Eaton, "Internet-Based Mental Health Interventions," *Mental Health Services Research*, Vol. 7, No. 2, June 2005, pp. 75–87.

Yen, S., M. E. Pagano, M. T. Shea, C. M. Grilo, J. G. Gunderson, A. E. Skodol, T. H. McGlashan, C. A. Sanislow, D. S. Bender, and M. C. Zanarini, "Recent Life Events Preceding Suicide Attempts in a Personality Disorder Sample: Findings from the Collaborative Longitudinal Personality Disorders Study," *Journal of Consulting and Clinical Psychology*, Vol. 73, No. 1, February 2005, pp. 99–105.

Zubin, J., and B. Spring, "Vulnerability: A New View of Schizophrenia," *Journal of Abnormal Psychology*, Vol. 86, No. 2, April 1977, pp. 103–126.